Miscommunication in Healthcare

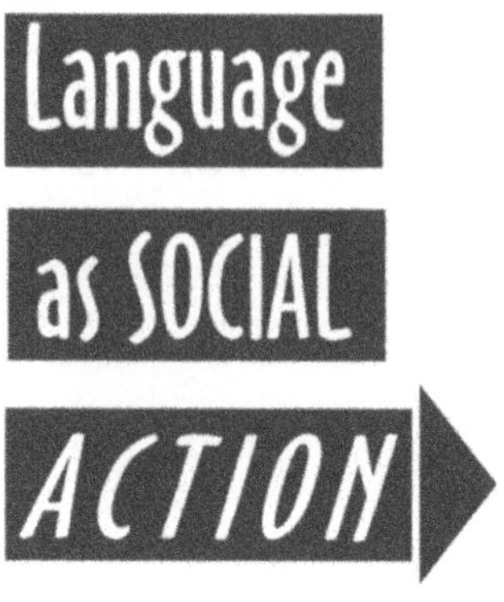

Howard Giles and David M. Markowitz
General Editors

Vol. 27

Bernadette M. Watson

Miscommunication in Healthcare

Solving a Wicked Problem

PETER LANG

New York · Berlin · Bruxelles · Chennai · Lausanne · Oxford

Bibliographic information published by the Deutsche Nationalbibliothek
The German National Library lists this publication in the German National Bibliography; detailed bibliographic data is available on the Internet at http://dnb.d-nb.de.

Library of Congress Cataloging-in-Publication Data

Names: Watson, Bernadette M. author
Title: Miscommunication in Healthcare : Solving a Wicked Problem / Bernadette M. Watson.
Description: New York : Peter Lang, 2026. | Series: Language as social action, 15292436 ; 27 | Includes bibliographical references and index. |
Identifiers: LCCN 2025047092 (print) | LCCN 2025047093 (ebook) | ISBN 9781636673783 hardback | ISBN 9781636673790 pdf | ISBN 9781636673806 epub
Subjects: LCSH: Communication in medicine | Health services administration--Patients
Classification: LCC R118 .W366 2026 (print) | LCC R118 (ebook) | DDC 610.14--dc23/eng/20260326
LC record available at https://lccn.loc.gov/2025047092
LC ebook record available at https://lccn.loc.gov/2025047093

Cover Image: Professor Bernadette M Watson PhD, MAPS, FHKAH and Yauheniya_Bandaruk and MdShohidul – stock.adobe.com

ISSN 1529-2436
ISBN 978-1-63667-378-3 (Print HB)
ISBN 978-3-0343-6493-5 (Print PB)
ISBN 978-1-63667-379-0 (ePDF)
ISBN 978-1-63667-380-6 (ePUB)
DOI 10.3726/b23563

Published by Peter Lang Publishing Inc., New York, USA

info@peterlang.com

This publication has been peer reviewed.

www.peterlang.com

Contact for General Product Safety Regulation (GPSR): gpsr@peterlang.com

In memory of Professor Cindy Gallois, my mentor, and Pamela Felton, my cousin, who was awarded the MBE for nursing services to the community of Oman.

Contents

Acknowledgements

I am indebted to my brother, Michael Jago, for his diligent and painstakingly careful editing of all drafts. Your help was indispensable.

Also to my husband, Geoffrey, who was always there for me and gave me the love and support I needed. Thank you both.

Finally, I want to thank David, Bernadette, Melanie, and Julie for being so generous with their contributions.

Using Intergroup Theory of Communication to Understand Healthcare Interactions

This book examines "health communication" from an "intergroup" perspective. Let me tell you first exactly what I mean by these two terms and how I shall be using them throughout this book. Health communication covers a huge area of research. It ranges from health promotion campaigns on posters in health clinics warning of the consequences of smoking or unhealthy diets, to TV ads about the dangers of alcohol abuse and the health risks of diabetes. It also includes information provided in leaflets or on websites, and in more detailed health manuals offering individuals guidance about better health choices. The scope is vast. In this book, I use the term "health communication" to relate specifically to how individuals communicate with each other when they engage in spoken, written and non-verbal exchanges about patient care. These exchanges may be between patients and health professionals, or professionals exchanging comments (written or spoken) with other professionals. I use the terms professional and provider interchangeably to represent any person who has undergone some kind of medical, nursing or health training and who works in a health context.

The second term is "intergroup". Chapter 2 will explain this in more detail, but I think it is worth reminding ourselves here that humans are essentially social animals who naturally form groups. These groups can be social or professional and will often represent an important part of a person's identity. Health professionals, such as doctors or nurses, identify very strongly with their particular profession and are proud of their membership. As we will see in Chapter 2, identifying with a group brings about a sense of self-worth and belonging. If a group is threatened, members will often rally to defend it. The same can be true of social groups. If a person is strongly aligned with one particular sporting team, they will support that team and want to see it succeed. Success makes the team supporter feel good about belonging to that social group. As social beings, we identify with like-minded people. I explain this more fully as we go through the chapters together, but it is important from the outset for me to make clear precisely what these two terms refer to within this book.

Authoring this book has been an exciting and fulfilling project for me. I spent some 30 years at The University of Queensland, Australia, where I was so fortunate to work with Cindy Gallois, Professor of Psychology, and it was with her guidance that I completed my PhD in health communication. But even before this, I had observed that individuals often changed their communication behaviour when interacting as patients with their doctors. People who were normally articulate and in control seemed to come away from their consultation without any real idea about what the doctor had said to them. I wondered why this was. Anxiety seemed to be one reason, and sometimes also the belief that the doctor knew best and that querying anything was somehow not allowed. When I began my research, it was apparent that patients would often blindly follow what the doctor had told them without any understanding of why a particular course of treatment had been recommended. Such a mindset has implications for patients not adhering to the recommended course of treatment, because they simply don't understand the rationale for it. Personal anxiety may also prevent a patient from volunteering critical information to the doctor. Patients usually know their own body better than anyone else, and remarks by a patient about their own observations are data that can assist the doctor in putting together the pieces of the particular health puzzle. The patient needs to feel able to voice their concerns and opinions. If they do not speak out for fear of raising matters that appear trivial, this too may be detrimental to health outcomes.

What became clear to me early on in my research was that health consultations are a very special type of interaction. Often, a patient may feel unable to express clearly what they want to say, leading to an unwillingness to communicate further with the doctor. Sometimes, the patient's perception that the doctor clearly possesses a higher societal status can negatively influence their ability to communicate assertively during a consultation. That doctors possess a high societal status is not a characteristic peculiar to Western culture. I also witnessed it when I moved to Hong Kong in 2016 to work at The Hong Kong Polytechnic University. The fact that there are such similarities between Western and Eastern cultures is an important aspect of health communication.

The importance of "role" in healthcare is paramount to understanding why health communication can be either effective or result in miscommunication. By "role" I am referring to the position that an individual holds within an institutional culture. For example, doctors and nurses are all individuals with their own personal likes and dislikes, but in a health setting, it is their professional position or "role" that is most important. It's perhaps worth adding that throughout this book, whenever I use the term doctor, I am referring to a medical doctor.

So much of healthcare communication research ignores the importance that group membership plays between speakers in a health context. Instead, health communication has focused on the personal attributes of each individual, describing encounters as interpersonal interactions. Minimal attention has been given to the fact that interactants can be viewed as members of specific groups such as doctors, patients or nurses. Often in healthcare encounters, this group membership is more prominent than an individual's personal likes and dislikes. The research examined in this book will clearly show that while encounters between individuals are indeed interpersonal at one level, more importantly, it is the group to which each individual belongs that carries most weight in the communication process. In essence, an individual's awareness of their group identity changes the communication dynamic, thereby reducing the relevance of the interpersonal dimension. This approach does not seek to ignore or deny personal identity, a unique combination of a person's characteristics, but when an individual enters healthcare contexts where they must communicate with others, it may, for a time, take a backseat. Human beings are social beings who generally thrive on interactions with others. In health interactions where social identity comes to the fore, personal idiosyncrasies become less prominent.

My first foray into health communication research focused on the patient's perspective and confirmed that the group identity of each speaker does indeed affect how they communicate. How this plays out is explored across the chapters of this book. Following on from patient-focused research, I became interested in how different health professionals communicated with each other. Health professionals are aware of the strong hierarchical structure that exists in healthcare, where doctors hold the highest status and power. Such a system has implications for how lower-status health disciplines interact with the higher-status doctors. For this reason, it seemed a natural and logical progression to expand my research interest to investigate how different health professional disciplines work together to negotiate and manage patient care and to assess the relative importance of their group identities. Just as with patient and doctor communication, health communication researchers were also ignoring the intergroup dynamic present when different health professionals work together.

What Does this Book Cover?

This book describes how health communication research has been conducted from the 1970s until the present day. In the beginning, research was predominantly atheoretical and interpersonal in focus, but over the last 30 years, a small number of health researchers have adopted an intergroup perspective in order to understand how communication plays out across a wide number of health situations and contexts. The chapters focus on how individuals negotiate and manage healthcare across this diverse range. I have concentrated on the research topics in healthcare with which I am most familiar. Communication accommodation theory (Giles, 2016; Giles et al., 2023) has been applied to several important health contexts, such as communication and ageing, intergenerational communication, and communication and physical disability. Each of these contexts can affect a person's well-being, and all are appropriate for examination in the health domain. However, while I'll draw on some literature in these domains where relevant, I can't possibly do justice to them all. Indeed, there are already many books dedicated to these topics, and the reader would be better informed by consulting these. I have provided a list of some seminal works for the interested reader at the end of this chapter.

A key challenge in writing an academic text is simply to make it interesting. The nature of such a text requires the author to focus on scholarship and research with a view to setting out the relevant theoretical concepts for scholars who may not be familiar with them, as well as expanding and critiquing theory for those academics more advanced. If successful, the text can inspire junior academics to investigate the theoretical framework further and provide those more advanced with new ways of using, refining, and expanding it. However, I have set myself a further challenge that, for me, is extremely important because it's so often ignored. I want health professionals who are not communication researchers and who are unfamiliar with the theoretical approach presented here to discover a different way of thinking about healthcare communication. From this new perspective, they may then explicitly recognise how the intergroup dynamics that exist in the healthcare context affect and shape communication behaviour. It's my experience that many health professionals implicitly intuit the intergroup environment in which they work and know that it influences such behaviour. But because health professionals are so embedded in the system, they see no alternatives and resign themselves to accepting the status quo. Health professionals are in a position to inform what researchers investigate, and new research directions can lead to changes for enhanced patient and health professional wellbeing. I hope the applied research described in this book will assist health professionals in finding new ways to improve rapport between patients and themselves, as well as with fellow professionals. This book may also provide new insights into how and why communication frequently fails.

So how can this book engage health professionals who live and breathe healthcare situations, and also be relevant to undergraduate and postgraduate communication scholars? When I began writing, I thought I could achieve a balance across these three audiences. But as I wrote, I realised something was not working. I could not make the book *come to life* if I kept it as a purely academic text. And, above all, I wanted health professionals to read it. I rethought it. I decided to promote this book as one that first and foremost engages health practitioners. This meant there would be less theory included in some chapters and a more applied focus overall. Of course, theory is necessarily woven into each chapter, and Chapter 2 is dedicated to explaining an intergroup approach. However, in my attempt to make the book transparently relevant and illustrate the different topics covered, each chapter will draw on actual health scenarios that directly speak to the chapter topic. Providing examples drawn from real-life health situations is the best way to illustrate the intergroup framework that drives this book. I have generally chosen examples that depict miscommunication because these bring home the message most clearly. There are also positive examples of excellent communication, though sadly, such events usually evaporate into the ether uncelebrated. Readers who work in healthcare will be able to assess the examples of miscommunication cited and compare them with their own experiences of events that went well as a result of effective communication. In this way, readers can break down sometimes complex theoretical concepts, linking them to personally experienced events. This should bring the theory to life for the student of health communication and, importantly, should allow health professionals to recall similar experiences and so judge whether this approach to health communication makes sense. My hope is that it will. This focus does not mean that communication academics will not benefit. I believe they will because they can appreciate how communication accommodation theory plays out in real-life scenarios.

Chapter Contents

Each chapter begins with a vignette (i.e., short scene) to illustrate its particular topic. I follow this with a statement about the key message of the chapter. At the end of the chapter, I reflect on what has been covered and ask the reader to consider their reaction to the content and, if they are a health practitioner, what they agree or disagree with and why. Have they gained any new insights into how healthcare operates at the current time?

Chapter 2 introduces the language and social psychology (LSP) approach to communication, leading to a discussion of communication accommodation theory (CAT). This CAT perspective places a person's group membership and its associated cultural norms centre stage in health encounters. One person is a patient, the other a health professional. Many health communication theories do not consider these two separate group identities. But recognition that there are two group memberships makes the encounter not just between two people (interpersonal) but rather between two groups (intergroup). This changes the communication dynamic. Finally, having laid out the theoretical framework of the LSP approach, I close by expanding on what this brings to the investigation of health communication research.

Chapter 3 marks the journey into more traditional topics. Spanning over 25 years of research, it is a longer chapter than others. It includes research into professionals from different health disciplines who interact with patients, patient carers, and parents of unwell children. I also highlight the work carried out in healthcare with parents in neonatal intensive care units (NICUs) and related special units.

Chapter 4 turns to issues surrounding interprofessional and interdisciplinary health communication and related multidisciplinary team interactions. I discuss the considerable amount of research by health communication scholars who have investigated how health professionals from different disciplines communicate with each other to manage patient care. Once again, in the past, there has been very little focus on the intergroup dynamics that drive such communication behaviour. This restricted view of communication as primarily interpersonal has created a serious gap, preventing a better understanding of how teams communicate across and within professions. Here, I critically review changes in undergraduate health-related university degree courses. Previously, university students across the different health disciplines followed separate curricula and did not interact. University programs now actively enable and encourage students from different health disciplines to share courses and learn together. Although this new focus takes education in the right direction, I discuss how the proposed changes often concentrate on communication competency purely as a skill. This narrow focus is at the expense of recognising how different health professions have their own medical language, cultural norms, and status, all of which must be considered when members interact as a multidisciplinary healthcare team.

In Chapter 5, another very important factor in healthcare is examined: intercultural communication. I describe how the presence of diverse global cultural values and beliefs influences the way health professionals from these different cultures communicate with each other and with their patients. I discuss research from a language and social psychology approach, investigating the challenges health professionals and patients face when they do not share the same first language. Difficulties in communication between individuals with different languages and cultures can be highly problematic for patient and health professional: their understanding of each other, the associated treatment regimen, and resultant patient safety. I also discuss how the presence of a mediator acting as interpreter is not without its own problems.

Chapter 6 brings together the complexity of health communication issues from a macro perspective. This is a logical place to position this chapter because it reflects on what we will have covered together thus far and poses key questions that will have emerged by then. Specifically, I explore the healthcare problems that occur in hospital settings. How does the organisational system and its associated institutional norms facilitate or hinder effective healthcare? Who can assist in solving these problems? What can be done to get a better grasp on healthcare miscommunication, adverse events, and tribal warfare? The chapter deliberately poses questions that demand urgent answers. I suggest that far more attention must be given to such questions in order to unpick and resolve the problems that healthcare currently faces.

Chapter 7 introduces the varied approaches that health communication researchers adopt when they apply CAT to health communication. It discusses the values and merits of both quantitative and qualitative data analysis and examines how combining these two approaches is a valuable technique for exploring research data. Applying mixed methods expands our understanding of both miscommunication and effective healthcare interactions. I discuss various approaches applied to measuring communication, including insider and outsider ratings, observations, simulations, and real-life interactions. I also unpack the challenges that researchers face when they embark on health communication research, which is often a lengthy process, requiring them to be sensitive to the demands and needs of the healthcare profession.

Chapter 8 explores what future directions should be taken in health communication research. Here, I discuss ways in which an intergroup perspective can be developed into an educational tool for health professionals to apply in their negotiations with patients and with other health professionals. I also introduce another theoretical approach that I have used in my own research ("positive psychology"), emphasising the positives that already exist in the healthcare system. I suggest focusing on what is done well (i.e., strengths), and not just on what goes wrong (i.e., weaknesses and failings). Strengths can certainly assist in reducing weaknesses and improving healthcare practice. I then discuss ways that I believe can improve collaboration between researchers and health professionals, leading to active change. Another important factor for future development is leadership and the roles that leaders can play in healthcare. Here, I deliberately focus on intergroup theory in the way that it relates to how leaders can work with others to enhance the health environment. I close the chapter with a discussion of online medical consultations and the relevance of intergroup theory to better manage them. They have been in existence for some time, and they demonstrate important differences from traditional face-to-face encounters, but since the COVID-19 pandemic, their frequency and acceptance have become far more prevalent.

And lastly, Chapter 9. Here I have invited three health practitioners, all of whom are familiar with intergroup theories of communication and with whom I have in the past collaborated, to explain why they see an intergroup perspective as critical to understanding the bigger picture of healthcare. Each comes from a different health discipline and brings their own unique perspective on why it is so important to recognise the existence of intergroup dynamics. David is a senior gastroenterologist who has worked both in Australia and the United States. Bernadette is a pharmacist who trained in Canada and then moved to Australia to study for her PhD. She has since returned to Canada to work. Mel has worked as an intensivist nurse in Australia and has also studied in Boston, USA. Each practitioner is well placed to offer their informed opinion. Following their comments, I turn to the patient perspective on health communication. I invited a friend who experienced a life-changing accident to discuss her experiences during her 18-month time as a hospital inpatient. Julie became a quadriplegic overnight and had to navigate an unknown and challenging environment as she adjusted to her new life. Taking up some of her observations, I show how an intergroup perspective explains some of the miscommunication she experienced. I conclude with some closing thoughts and express the hope that I have opened new and exciting avenues for all readers of this book.

Further Reading

Harwood, J. (2019). *Language, communication, and intergroup relations: A celebration of the scholarship of Howard Giles* (1 ed.). Routledge. <https://doi.org/10.4324/9781315142807>

Hummert, M. L., & Nussbaum, J. F. (2001). *Aging, communication, and health : Linking research and practice for successful aging.* Lawrence Erlbaum Associates.

The Importance of Identity in Healthcare Contexts

A colleague and I were presenting a workshop to nursing, medical and allied health students. Our purpose was to discuss with the audience how a person's health discipline defined the way they communicated with their colleagues in both their own particular health field and other health areas. The students unknowingly made this task very easy for us. As each student entered the lecture room, they looked around and then headed for a seat of their choice. When everyone had arrived, my colleague and I looked at our audience: each student had chosen to sit near someone from their own profession. Students from medicine, nursing, physical therapy, occupational therapy and other represented professions had all grouped themselves with those they identified with. It was as if we had colour-coded the seating by profession and asked each person to sit with their own group. Now this phenomenon is not unique to health professions, but it clearly demonstrates how individuals are drawn to gather together in groups where they feel similar.

The scene I describe occurred some years ago when I was involved in running some workshops at a Brisbane hospital. It shows how we connect with our groups and form relationships. This chapter explains how our relationships with others are often exceedingly complex. In any one conversation, our attitudes and reactions to a person can fluctuate considerably. Understanding exactly how this happens can enable us to manage future relationships more effectively.

I use a language and social psychology (LSP) approach to the study of health communication. In this chapter, I shall introduce CAT (Giles et al., 1987; Watson et al., 2016), a dynamic and highly effective theory within LSP that, in various forms, has been applied to health communication for over 30 years. While communication scholars familiar with its concepts may wish to skim or even skip this chapter, other readers less familiar with this content will find it not only invaluable in itself but also essential in order to fully appreciate subsequent chapters. It presents the background necessary for understanding an LSP perspective, and it introduces ways in which the application of CAT provides insights into how individuals communicate with one another across many existing health contexts.

We know that human beings are highly complex creatures who are also individually unique. To better understand the complexities of communication within any health interaction, we would be well-advised to utilise more than one theoretical perspective. My aim is to establish the importance of examining group dynamics within such interactions and so reveal how an individual's identification with a group can influence their communication behaviour. For many people, visiting a health professional, being a hospital inpatient, or visiting someone in hospital can be discomforting and often frightening. Most patients naturally look to the knowledge and expertise of their health provider, and it is this seeking of expertise that makes a two-way health interaction very different from a social chat with a colleague (see Chapter 3). For health professionals, the health context is their normal daily life, which they must negotiate and manage. However, we will see, for instance, that encounters of some junior staff with health colleagues can be daunting and can challenge their ability to put forward their own opinions about a patient's care (see Chapter 4). Patients and health professionals alike have roles to play that reflect their group identities and which go beyond who they are as individuals. Conforming to a social norm or role is a part of the health context and must be included in the complex communicative puzzle.

Understanding Language and Social Psychology

An LSP approach explores how our attitudes to social phenomena influence our communication behaviours with individuals, groups, institutions, policy makers and so forth. LSP researchers therefore focus on intrapersonal, interpersonal and intergroup communication to assess people's beliefs, values and attitudes. In this book, I will need to refer to both the person who is the current speaker and to the person who responds. There are many terms that can be used to describe these two persons. Because this book has a broad readership of not only communication scholars but also health professionals and others interested in health communication, I will use two simple terms. Unless specifically identified, the person speaking or initiating a conversation with another will be termed the speaker; the person being addressed will be termed the speech partner.

In a health context, an LSP approach explores how patients, health professionals from different disciplines, as well as health carers such as family members, differ in their communication behaviour when they interact with one another. As a typical example, when a nurse discusses patient care with a patient, they will generally use a different communication style from the one adopted when discussing that patient with another health professional. An LSP perspective seeks to make explicit the reasoning ("cognitions") and aims ("motivations") that shape communication behaviour during interaction. The cognitions and motivations that drive a nurse's communication style when with a patient will normally be based on their belief that the patient is a layperson without any knowledge of medical terminology (nurse's cognition). They will simply want the patient to understand clearly what is being explained to them (nurse's motivation). In contrast, the nurse's communication style will differ when speaking to a health professional who is, say, a physiotherapist. In this instance, the nurse's change in behaviour will be based on the belief that the physiotherapist is fully conversant with the relevant terminology (cognition), and accordingly, they will use such technical language as is appropriate to explain the patient's treatment needs (motivation). A further motivation for the nurse may be a wish to appear knowledgeable and competent. In any situation, more than one motivation may be present.

This example may seem straightforward, but communication can so easily go wrong. The nurse, believing the patient a layperson, will have used simple language to explain the treatment details. However, this may well annoy the patient if they too happen to be a trained nurse. The patient will then not be satisfied with everyday language and will require more relevant medical terminology. If the patient reveals that they are medically qualified, the nurse will likely reassess their cognition about the patient and decide that more technical language is appropriate. But the nurse's motivation remains the same: they still want the patient to have a clear understanding of their health condition. The nurse rectifies the situation by altering their word choice to match the perceived comprehension level of the patient. However, the nurse's interaction with the physiotherapist may not be so simple to fix if that goes wrong.

Nurses and physiotherapists are educated within their separate professions to attain their respective qualifications. In learning different techniques, each profession will often use dissimilar medical terms reflecting their separate disciplines. Thus, the nurse may assume incorrectly that the medical terms they've used have been understood by the physiotherapist. In response, the physiotherapist could admit to unfamiliarity with these terms and request some clarification. But if the physiotherapist is new and very junior and the nurse is very senior, the physiotherapist may decide to hide their unfamiliarity for fear of looking incompetent. They may reason that they can research the terms later. This interaction will not have been so successful because the physiotherapist is motivated to appear competent at the expense of ensuring adequate comprehension. Using an LSP approach can assist in uncovering why conversations go well and why they go badly. In healthcare, this is often complex (see Chapter 4).

Yet another version of the above scenario is possible. The nurse may believe they have used everyday language with the patient, but may also inadvertently have included some jargon. This is no problem for the patient who is also a nurse, but for the non-medical patient, it will almost certainly cause a degree of difficulty in understanding. The nurse's cognitions and motivations remain as described above, but now their choice of language is, in part, unintentionally inappropriate. In the same way as the physiotherapist wouldn't admit to not understanding the nurse, the patient may not want to appear ignorant and so may not query any medical terms. This is not a good outcome for the patient. The take-home message from this last scenario is significant: how a person believes they are communicating and how they are actually communicating may be discordant. In an ideal world, there would be perfect concord between what a person says and does and the perception of this communicative behaviour by others. This book will demonstrate that such an agreement does not always hold true.

An Overview of Speech Accommodation Theory

Drawing on social psychology, Howard Giles first developed speech accommodation theory (Giles, 1973). He (see Giles & Powesland, 1975) integrated four seminal theories into speech accommodation theory (SAT) so as to more fully explain communication encounters. These theories were social identity theory (Tajfel, 1978), similarity attraction theory (Byrne, 1969), attribution theory (Heider, 1958) and social exchange theory (Homans, 1961). Each theory provides insights into how and why people behave when they communicate with others. As we shall see, SAT was later expanded to become CAT.

Giles developed SAT in the 1970s and originally focused on accent mobility: the ways in which a person can alter their speech when interacting with others. Modifications to personal accent, pitch, tone, speech rate and volume he termed "approximation". He next identified four types of speech behaviour. The first, linguistic convergence, occurs when a person produces speech more similar to their speech partner. Conversely, the second, linguistic divergence, occurs when a speaker changes their speech to sound less similar to their speech partner. Maintenance, the third behaviour, occurs when a speaker does not alter their speech at all. This is now normally judged as a form of divergence, because the speaker is making no effort to change their speech in order either to emulate or to distinguish themselves from their speech partner. In the fourth behaviour, complementarity, the speaker does alter their speech to be less similar to their speech partner, but unlike divergence, the behaviour is adopted in order to facilitate conversation. An example would be an agitated patient in the hospital emergency department shouting or speaking too quickly to the treating clinician. One solution would be for the health professional to speak softly and slowly in order to defuse the situation and calm the patient. Complementarity is accommodative behaviour because, although divergent, the health professional's goal is to improve the encounter for the patient.

To explain variations in speech production between groups, Giles turned to social identity theory; as a social psychologist, he recognised that other psychological processes can influence the communication behaviour of the complex human being. Social identity theory, commonly abbreviated to SIT (Tajfel, 1979), emphasises the importance that individuals place on their particular group memberships, of which there may be many. These include, but are not limited to, affiliation through nationality, gender, religion, political beliefs, sports and professions. When individuals converse with others, it is often the group membership most dominant in that interaction that influences communication exchanges. SIT examines how a person's perceptions about the group membership of their speech partner can influence their communication production with that person. It is key to Giles' SAT and the later expanded CAT. Tajfel developed SIT to investigate why individuals discriminate against some groups yet favour others. His research evolved from his experiences as a Polish Jew during the Second World War. He had observed that those Germans who identified themselves as Nazis subjected Jewish people to appalling and inhumane treatment; he wanted to understand the mechanisms at work which would explain their dehumanisation of a specific societal group.

SIT is a complex theory of intergroup behaviour; it proposes that individuals possess two categories of identity. The first is their personal identity, comprising their unique likes and dislikes – their idiosyncrasies – such as enjoying novels and disliking celery. The second is their social or group identity. Individuals can belong to any number of groups; the number and importance will vary for each person. However, in SIT, Tajfel postulates that often when an individual interacts with another, it is their allegiance to a particular social group that is more important than their personal identity. As a typical example from a health context, in assessing a hospital inpatient's treatment plan, two doctors will perceive their shared professional group identity as far more important than other interpersonal characteristics, such as enjoying long-distance hikes with their walking club. The latter is not relevant to the immediate context.

Over the years, many psychologists have conducted experiments to replicate ingroup favouritism and outgroup discrimination (e.g., Brewer & Kramer, 1985;

Otten, 2016). Findings consistently confirm that individuals are social beings who place great importance and value on their own ingroup memberships but may often place less value on outgroups. Why should this be? One reason is that individuals identify with and feel positively disposed towards their own groups. This sense of belonging frequently brings with it a feeling of self-worth. Individuals perceive they share the same beliefs that bind them with other ingroup members. Membership becomes a valued part of who they are. By contrast, ingroup members often do not value the beliefs of outgroup members; they favour their ingroup and discriminate against those with an outgroup allegiance. However, although SIT concerns itself with behaviours of favouritism and discrimination associated with group membership, it does not take into account how ingroup and outgroup bias translates into communication behaviour. For further information on SIT, see the bibliography at the end of this chapter.

The second theory that Giles drew on was similarity attraction theory. Byrne (1969) postulated that individuals feel attracted to people they perceive as being similar to themselves. The connection between this assumption and SIT is immediately clear. Ingroup members perceive similarities between themselves, which they value highly, but in outgroups, they often perceive differences that they don't especially value. Giles proposed that individuals interact differently depending on whether they are with people they sense are similar or with people having no apparent common link. However, a person who is not an ingroup member, but who has aspirations to become one, may strive to appear more similar to a member of that particular group. They may wish to be liked by the outgroup member so that, in time, they may pass into the outgroup which then becomes the ingroup. Cultivating the necessary characteristics associated with a particular group may enhance the chances of an individual joining that group. Someone trained as a nurse may desire more responsibility and want to study further to become a doctor. As they plan their transition to medical school, it's very probable that the nurse will wish to be seen positively by doctors. They may also be less likely to criticise doctors while they aspire to join this group.

The third addition informing SAT, attribution theory (Heider, 1958), explains how individuals attribute meaning to their own and others' behaviour. Speakers who perceive their speech partner as unfriendly or unhelpful can consider this behaviour as either intentional or unintentional. A person perceiving their speech partner's behaviour as deliberately unhelpful and believing it to be within their control to behave differently, will most likely judge them more negatively than if they viewed that behaviour as not being under their full volition or control. The latter judgement would imply that the perceived unhelpful behaviour must be attributed to other causes. As an example, a hospital inpatient may want to spend time talking to a nurse who is on a medication round. If the nurse gives only short responses and does not stay to chat, the patient may feel this to be unfriendly. On the other hand, the patient may realise that the nurse has a large number of patients requiring the correct medicines and looks tired. In that case, the patient may be more forgiving of the nurse's lack of engagement.

Social exchange theory (Homans, 1961), the fourth component of SAT, predicts that individuals seek to maximise rewards and minimise costs. Giles et al. (1977) argued that this theory was relevant in further explaining an individual's use of linguistic convergence and divergence. Specifically, if a person believes that the rewards of speech convergence will outweigh the costs incurred by the effort of physically converging, then convergence is likely to occur. Alternatively, costs could outweigh benefits. For example, if the likely reward for a speaker linguistically converging is a high approval rating from their speech partner, but only at the cost of losing their own sense of individuality (e.g., not standing up for rights they believe in), then the speaker may decide that the cost of convergence is too high a price to pay. Sometimes this occurs subconsciously. Furthermore, not everyone has the same potential linguistic repertoire. Some have a gift for copying the speech characteristics of others; some simply don't. In summary, SAT sought to explain how individuals may have many motives for altering their speech so as to converge to or diverge from that of their speech partner; some motives may be conscious, some not.

From SAT to CAT

In the 1980s, SAT was further expanded to encompass other aspects of communication. Nikolas Coupland and colleagues introduced three communication strategies which ultimately led to SAT being renamed CAT (Coupland et al., 1988). SAT was becoming far more wide-ranging and comprehensive in scope; its revised name reflected this development. These new strategies described communication behaviours that explored other specific linguistic and non-linguistic strategies that a person might adopt in an interaction. Gallois et al. (1995) used the term "sociolinguistic strategies" to describe these additions. The first, *interpretability*, concerns a speaker's attention to their speech partner's communicative competence. A speaker using complicated words or jargon that their speech partner will not comprehend is demonstrating non-accommodative interpretability, for example, a health provider using medical jargon when speaking to a medically untrained patient. Conversely, a simpler word choice, ensuring that a patient clearly understands the content, is accommodative. But if the choice of wording is oversimplified, this too will be non-accommodative, as it may be judged by the patient as patronising.

The second new strategy, *discourse management*, concerns the interaction process or *conversational needs* of a speaker rather than the particular content. Effective discourse management by the speech partner demonstrates that the speaker is being positively attended to during the conversation. Nonverbal gestures such as nodding the head, making eye contact and leaning forward to show attentiveness would demonstrate this, as would simple verbal behaviours such as back-channelling (i.e., responding with an "uh-huh" or "mm-hmm"). A health provider who listens attentively to a patient and prompts for more information is applying accommodative discourse management. The opposite is true if the provider does not maintain eye contact, appears distracted or does not encourage the patient to speak.

The third additional strategy, *interpersonal control*, concerns the role relations of the two persons and the extent to which the current speaker is constrained by the group membership most salient (i.e., dominant) to them. A health provider may wish to control a consultation by asking closed questions that don't allow the patient to expand on their responses. A doctor may interrupt the patient, abruptly change the topic or terminate the conversation when they decide they have enough information. These behaviours can constrain the patient's communication and lead to their passivity, the patient coming to play a less than equal role in the consultation. In contrast, a health provider who sees their patient as equal in the encounter may adopt open-ended questions, encourage input and welcome any queries the patient may have. Accommodative interpersonal control enables the patient to have some say in the consultation and demonstrates a more even balance in status.

Subsequently, one further strategy, *emotional expression*, was introduced to take account of the emotional needs of speakers within an interaction (Watson & Gallois, 1998; Williams et al., 1990). A speaker who shows concern and provides reassurance and support when needed is demonstrating an accommodative emotional expression. Such behaviour acknowledges the other's anxiety and worries. This particular strategy has been shown as highly important in consultations between health providers and patients; it can predict patient satisfaction alongside a patient's intention to adhere to treatment (Watson & Gallois, 2004). Perhaps unsurprisingly, emotional expression is also important in interprofessional interactions (see Chapter 4).

Thus far, the application of CAT to predict, reveal and examine motives for communication behaviours has been described in outline. CAT is both a general theory of communication and one tailored to explain communication across specific contexts. Several variations of a CAT model have been developed, but they all follow each speaker's experiences in turn from the beginning of an interaction to its conclusion. CAT shows how one or both speakers may alter their attitude towards the other during the course of an interaction. It also allows the researcher to examine the subsequent evaluation of the interaction experience by the participants. As this book is concerned with health communication, examples to explain the model will be set within the health context.

A final but no less important feature of CAT is its potential for demonstrating the relationship between an individual's interpersonal and intergroup identities. This relationship is fluid: each identity can vary to a greater or lesser extent, but at any one moment only one can be salient.

I've been emphasising the importance of group identity in the health context and that CAT, unlike other communication theories, can explicitly recognise this. I've also stated that CAT doesn't deny the importance of an individual's personal identity, but rather that it demonstrates within many contexts that this identity is not always the salient one. How one identity can take prominence during an interaction needs some further elaboration before we move on to the next chapter. So, let's look at four contrasting scenarios, in each of which two individuals are interacting.

(1) A medical consultant (i.e., a senior doctor) and a senior nurse are on a hospital ward discussing a patient's treatment. They do not know each other in any capacity other than as healthcare professionals. In this interaction, the professional identity of each is highly salient as it is these particular clinical disciplines that are important during the interaction. Their interpersonal identities are not relevant. This is typical of most health professional encounters – they are high intergroup and low interpersonal interactions.

(2) A husband (a cardiologist) and wife (a surgeon) are discussing a film they have just watched and how much they enjoyed it. In this interaction, their personal identities are highly salient as they are focused on each other as close individuals who have enjoyed a film. Their professional group identities are unimportant, and so their interaction represents one of high interpersonal salience but low intergroup importance. How could their identities change to one of high intergroup importance? In the following way.

Both are still thinking about the film when the husband abruptly changes the subject and makes a general but slightly negative comment about surgeons. In response, the wife feels that her own ingroup, surgeons, is being threatened, and so her professional identity becomes the more important. At this moment, she sees her husband primarily in his professional role. It's very possible that the husband doesn't realise that he's changed the interaction dynamic from high interpersonal for both to one in which his wife sees him predominantly in his cardiologist role. At this moment, he is still focusing on them as a couple.

However, his wife's manner and communication behaviour will signal that she is now interacting with him as a professional. His reaction may well be to focus on his own professional identity, and the interaction will change to one that has high intergroup salience for them both. This illustrates how we alter our identity and the way we communicate with each other according to the immediate context. Note that at any one time, only one identity can be salient for each person.

(3) A pharmacy assistant is serving a customer; they have never met before. Neither their intergroup nor their interpersonal identities, therefore, matter. It is quite a neutral situation – their interpersonal and intergroup identities are of low importance: neither is salient.

(4) While working together in the Human Relations Department of a hospital, two friends are chatting about an upcoming holiday. Here, their personal identities as two individuals with likes and dislikes are important; any group identities are irrelevant. This interaction demonstrates high interpersonal but low intergroup importance.

In these scenarios, I've illustrated how context influences whether an individual's personal or group identity comes to the fore. Communication is an endlessly dynamic process; it is not inflexibly static. CAT allows identification of shifts in goals and identities during any interaction. When a speaker changes the focus (effectively the context) of a conversation, this in turn can change what is salient to their speech partner, and consequently the latter's attitudes and communication behaviours. In scenario 2, I chose to illustrate how even high interpersonal salience can change quite easily because of the relationship between two people.

Review

An LSP approach endeavours to reveal motives in human communication behaviour by applying perspectives from social psychology. CAT exemplifies an LSP perspective because its goal is not just to explain why particular communication behaviours occur, but also predict the likelihood of such behaviours recurring in similar situations. Some critics have argued that CAT is unwieldy and overly complex (see: Gallois et al., 2018). Nonetheless, it has repeatedly shown itself to be a robust theory capable of offering insightful explanations for miscommunication. Its application has made important advances in better explaining the mechanisms that underpin interactions. As later chapters will show, CAT has become an effective educational tool in reducing communication failure. Applying CAT in the health sector is creating a better understanding of how miscommunication occurs and of what actions can be taken to improve communication between patients and health professionals and between health professionals themselves.

This chapter has covered the key philosophy that underpins CAT. It has explained why CAT is an extremely useful reference tool for those seeking to understand effective communication as well as miscommunication in healthcare. The following chapters investigate many domains within healthcare interactions, drawing on an LSP approach but especially on CAT as a robust theory that can predict, unpack and explain communication behaviour. In Chapter 3, we look at the heartland of health communication: interactions between patients and their health providers. We'll see that the power distance between a health provider and the patient is dynamic and can change within a consultation. We will also see that the patient's perception of their role as patient, and the health provider's perception as the clinician, can dictate the way such an encounter unfolds.

Some Personal Review Points

I hope you have now gained new insights into why your communication behaviour can fluctuate in any one conversation.

- Can you think of an occasion when you switched from seeing someone primarily in their professional role to seeing them in a more personal way?
- By the end of that same conversation, did you revert to seeing them again in their professional role?
- What are your thoughts about this? Did your reactions to your speech partner change as your view of their role changed?

Further Reading

Brown, R. (2020). The social identity approach: Appraising the Tajfellian legacy. *British Journal of Social Psychology*, *59*(1), 5–25. <https://doi.org/10.1111/bjso.12349>

Tajfel, H., & Turner, J. C. (1986). The social identity theory of intergroup behavior. In S. Worchel & W. G. Austin (Eds.), *Psychology and intergroup relations* (pp. 7–24). Nelson-Hall.

Health Communication Between Health Providers and Patients

What do doctors believe makes for an effective medical consultation? Here in this recorded extract is what one doctor (a general practitioner with 21 years' experience) told me:

I think the development of a personal relationship with a patient is critical and seeing them more as friends rather than patients. It is a very different sort of professional role as far as I can see – or professional relationship. I know a number of my colleagues would probably feel a bit uncomfortable with that. And it might also reflect on the type of patients I end up seeing, but a lot of them I have seen for a very long time. A lot of them have a lot of problems and pretty rocky journeys along life and sometimes what you offer them is – we can't give them a pill, or you can't give them a simple formula for solving the problem. So, you act as someone who travels the journey with them, and over a period of time you develop very close relationships with them. So, of course, that requires respect, so that is I think a critical thing. And developing that means you've got to find out about them as people, you've got to understand their family background and what they do, the things they like over a period of time. You build up a pretty strong picture of the individual you're dealing with.

To me, this demonstrates the delicate balance required between intergroup and interpersonal communication in health provider and patient consultations. Finding and maintaining that balance is by no means easy.

Review of Communication Between Health Professionals and Patients

Health provider and patient communication research has been prolific since the 1970s (Korsch et al., 1968; Korsch & Negrete, 1972; Pendleton, 1983). Why has it been such an intensive area of research? Health practitioners and communication researchers now recognise that effective communication between health professionals and their patients is essential for achieving positive patient outcomes. Adherence to treatment, for example, requires good communication (Burgoon et al., 1990; Ley, 1988). When patients understand and follow their treatment regimen, they are more likely to experience beneficial outcomes (e.g. Bennett et al., 2011). In this chapter, I'll briefly discuss health communication research as it has traditionally been conducted; I'll then introduce research that uses an intergroup perspective. I'll concentrate first on doctor and patient interactions, as this topic makes up much of health communication research. I'll go on to examine some work on nurse and patient interactions and will also review research on interactions between other types of health professionals and patients. I'll include some work that has been conducted on what is known as "futile care", because this particular topic highlights difficulties facing health providers when trying to manage end-of-life care for their patients. Here, by adopting a language and social psychology perspective, we can gain insights into the motivations that underlie the health providers' recommended treatment.

Approaches to Early Research

It's true to say that much of the early research into health provider and patient interactions was atheoretical (Freimuth et al., 2006; Thompson & Robinson, 2021). For many researchers, including myself, atheoretical research can be highly problematic. Researchers from some communication disciplines may not necessarily view this as a research concern, and it's true that anecdotal data are interesting and provide many insights into the health domain. But from my own psychology perspective, it is questionable how much we can make sense of anecdotal data and gain insights into why specific behaviours are adopted if we don't invoke a theoretical framework (see Chapter 2).

From a social psychology stance, it's crucial to pose clear research questions in order to drive how data are collected and analysed. To derive appropriate research questions, psychology demands theory. Without theory, it isn't possible to predict or explain findings from the data collected. However, it isn't the case that early research into health consultations was not well executed. For example, health researchers often examined the words that doctors used in responding to their patients. Bales' interaction process was an early form of analysis employed to clearly describe and code these responses into 12 categories (Bales, 1950). Such coding is a sound procedure, but it can only describe, not explain, why doctors speak as they do. Theory is needed for the development of predictions. Length of consultations was another topic of interest in early research. It was argued that doctors who spent longer in consultations would be viewed more positively by their patients. This turned out not to be always the case. Korsch and Negrete (1972) found that longer consultations could sometimes result in reduced patient satisfaction. These conflicting findings indicate that observing and describing behaviour in consultations, although interesting, is insufficient if the researcher's goal is to gain insights from the data that will enable the prediction of what will be effective for the patient and what will not. What matters in studying long and short consultations is the actual communication process. Specifically, what occurs during a consultation is more important than the length of the consultation.

Applying a theory to understand the actual process is a separate endeavour from applying a detailed analysis system such as Bales' interaction process analysis or the Roter interaction analysis system (RIAS: Roter & Larson, 2002). Researchers sometimes become annoyed when accused of being atheoretical; they argue that they've invested a great deal of thought and energy into carefully coding their data for detailed analysis. Rigorous coding provides a systematic and detailed description of the data. But, in psychology, coding is only one step, albeit a critical one, in the research design (see Chapter 7). We must delve more deeply and ask questions. How can this detailed information explain why the interaction was perceived as positive (by the patient or by the health professional)? Using empirical evidence from previous observations, can we predict when an interaction is no longer going well? How can we observe and understand the processes that underlie the interactants' communication behaviours and their assessment of the consultation? For those researchers who take an LSP perspective, such questions are of paramount importance.

The role of communication skills was another topic examined during the late twentieth century. Much of the research focused on the design of training interventions for doctors in order to improve their skills. Cegala and Broz (2002, 2003) reviewed 26 representative studies from the literature on physician communication training published between 1990 and 2001. Their review uncovered serious gaps in the research literature, such as insufficient detail in the method section of the papers. They noted that studies were inconsistent both in their definition of communication skills and in the assessment of these skills by the variety of methods employed. Notwithstanding the many serious methodological deficiencies, they were able to state that, in broad terms, the training showed some success, but they criticised the fact that few studies assessed the long-term retention of skills.

In their 2003 book chapter, they also reviewed 19 studies on the teaching of communication skills to patients, remarking that little research had been carried out in this area. They found that the focus was largely on information exchange skills, a description they found simplistic and over-generalised, and which they believed obscured the important separate aspects of seeking, providing, and verifying (i.e., checking) information. The majority of research concentrated on the first of these aspects, particularly through question asking, yet the effect of training was "moderate, at best" (Cegala & Broz, 2003, p.105). Little attention was given to the specific concerns – the content – of the patients' questions. Methodologically, question asking was too broad a term to be useful, while other ways of seeking information were largely overlooked. Where the training intervention involved role modelling or practice, results from post-training demonstrated improvement in patients' communication behaviour.

As Cegala and Broz stated, "Most patients benefit from, indeed require, seeing someone model these behaviours, and afterwards they need the opportunity to practice the skills, ideally with feedback" (2003 p. 112). However, they recognised that for most clinical practices the cost of this kind of patient education is prohibitive, and they recommended that future research should address this challenging situation. As none of the patient training interventions looked at long-term changes in behaviour, the ability of patients to transfer skills when interacting with different health providers remains unknown.

Viewing this research from an LSP approach, it matters that no attention was given to the communication dynamics between the interactants, or to other patient characteristics such as gender, age and sociocultural background. Where was the theoretical framework that would inform the studies beyond simply measuring communication behaviour and possible changes? As I argue in Chapter 4, communication skills do matter, but by themselves, these are insufficiently illuminating without attention to the intergroup dynamics of the situation and the particular context.

Doctor and Patient Communication – Early Research

In investigating health provider and patient interactions, the dominant approach was, and in the majority of studies still is, to see them as interpersonal in nature. Whether physically face to face or merely virtual, they do possess an interpersonal component, but they also contain elements that are not interpersonal. Viewing these encounters as intergroup can give additional insights into the whole consultation process (see Chapter 2), in which the intergroup component is often a stronger driver of the interaction dynamic than the interpersonal. However, its importance in medical interactions has not been widely accepted (see: Brann et al., 2021). As a case in point, Harrington et al. (2022) provide a comprehensive chapter on theoretical and methodological issues in health communication research, highlighting the interdisciplinary nature of this domain. They discuss interpersonal, mass and mass-personal communication but do not consider intergroup communication. Failure to recognise the status and power differentials that exist between health providers and patients, or to consider the importance of roles and of cultural and societal norms in such interactions, is to miss vital information.

Over thirty years ago, Street and Wiemann (1988) acknowledged the uniqueness of the physician–patient relationship,[1] highlighting the "professional" aspect of the medical interaction and emphasising the intergroup rather than interpersonal dimension. They argued that these dyadic exchanges are professional encounters, and that the health provider and patient consultation is not an interpersonal interaction. Further, they stated that many health professionals often prefer to emphasise their professional role in their communication style. This may mean that they remain socially distant, a style that some patients actually prefer (Burgoon et al., 1987). Burgoon et al. also found, however, that patients are positively responsive to physicians who are more interpersonal in their communication style (that is, show warmth and involvement, concern, liking, responsiveness, etc.). These contradictory findings indicate that doctors and patients may have different expectations about how each should typically behave during a consultation.

Street Jnr and Buller (1988) investigated nonverbal communication between doctors and patients, finding a significant difference for doctors in their style of interaction with highly anxious and with less anxious patients. When dealing with more anxious patients, doctors used less physical touch and adjusted their turn-taking to encourage the patients to talk. Street Jnr and Buller also found that doctors tended to match some behaviours of older patients more closely than those of younger patients, but matched pause and response latencies (i.e., delays in replying) more evenly with first-time patients. The matching or mirroring of patient behaviours demonstrates that doctors are focused on the immediate interaction. This is an indicator of empathy and liking by the doctor. Such behaviours have been correlated with patient satisfaction (Larsen & Smith, 1981). Street (1993) argued that communication behaviours should not be isolated from the meaning that led to their use, or the context in which they occurred. In other words, interactions should be investigated holistically; otherwise, the

1 I use the terms doctor and physician interchangeably to refer to the same profession. In the United States, the term physician is often used more than doctor, but in other parts of the world (e.g., Australia and the United Kingdom), doctor is more common.

validity of results obtained in isolation is questionable. Rather than analysing specific channels of communication, researchers should adopt a more functional approach to studying behaviour. He argued for an examination of entire sections of communication with all its related behaviours.

Although this approach would necessitate small chunks of behaviour being examined over an entire consultation, these chunks might include more valid data (but see Capella & Street, 1985; Street, 1985 for a critique of the functional approach). In addition, Buller and Street Jnr (1992) and Street (1992) argued that the reciprocal nature of the interaction between health providers and patients demands that both interactants be investigated. Recognising that a consultation has its own specific parameters is critical to investigating and understanding the communication process that occurs during each medical encounter. There is also a more general consideration that many scholars do not take into account: any interaction is by definition a two-way process with each interactant influencing the other. An LSP approach recognises this two-way dynamic as well as the context in which it occurs.

In some early studies, patient satisfaction measures were used to evaluate the relative success of such medical encounters (Ley, 1988; Schneider & Tucker, 1992). Just how might a patient assess a consultation? Factors they might consider would include the extent to which they perceive the doctor as listening to them, recognising what the symptoms they describe suggest is the problem, explaining this to them, providing a clear treatment regimen, and showing appropriate interest and concern. Patient satisfaction, as a key indicator of whether a consultation has been successful, is still frequently used, but given the broad scope of what it can cover, I don't believe it should be the only measure. Some recent research that Dr Susan Baker and I have undertaken shows that a patient may be dissatisfied with a consultation when they request a specific type of medication which a doctor refuses (Baker & Watson 2025). Of course, the doctor may be absolutely correct in their judgement that the requested drug is not in the best interests of their patient. However, it can result in the patient giving a low satisfaction score for that particular doctor. Nonetheless, patient satisfaction is still a standard measure used in health communication research, and it remains important. Such other measures of the patient's perceptions should also be included for a more balanced picture of the consultation.

Street (1991) was one of the first researchers to review the role of accommodation in medical consultations and to advocate effective communication between doctors and patients as being essential for good healthcare delivery. For Street, the role of accommodation was central to health consultations. Since his chapter, a great deal of research has explored accommodative stance by health providers, but Street emphasised the importance of CAT in the doctor and patient domain. He cited two key reasons that need to be at the forefront to ensure effective doctor-patient consultations. Firstly, the talk that occurs between the patient and doctor is critical for understanding the patient's health issues. Street recognised that patient characteristics could shape the consultation trajectory and affect the necessity to explore the actual talk during the consultation. With technological developments, less communication may be required for accurate diagnoses – even more so today than in 1991 – but talk is still a very important part of the interaction. Secondly, Street emphasised what he called the affective component of the doctor and patient partnership, because this assists rapport building and engagement by the patient.

Watson and Gallois (1998) established that although patients were satisfied with health professionals who presented with low levels of affect (i.e., mood) and were strictly task focused, they were more positive when a health professional demonstrated levels of interpersonal interest and concern. This was shown in the significantly higher scores for patients on three scales: satisfaction, evaluation of effectiveness, and likelihood to return to that health professional for a further consultation. Street's chapter paved the way for future research that promoted the wider use of CAT in health communication. As an example, D'Agostino and Bylund (2011) developed the nonverbal accommodation analysis system, highlighting the often less researched aspect of nonverbal communication. Their coding system was greatly influenced by CAT, thus bringing together coding and a theory to explain and predict communication behaviour.

As noted above, the term health provider in health research literature has more often than not referred only to the doctor. This is still true in the current period. For example, the recent new edition of the Oxford University Press text "Communicating about health" (Du Pre & Cook Overton, 2023) and the most recent Handbook by Routledge on health communication (Thompson & Harrington, 2022) both have sections on communication between health providers and patients. These sections focus on doctors at the expense of other health professionals. In addition, they maintain an interpersonal perspective even when issues around power differentials are noted (see Chapter 3 Du Pre & Cook Overton, 2023, pp. 39–40).

In contrast, this book promotes the importance of including an intergroup perspective when investigating health communication. Accordingly, the remainder of this chapter is devoted to research into health provider and patient communication that has adopted an intergroup approach. Health providers other than doctors are included. This intergroup perspective extends beyond CAT and includes the theory of willingness to communicate (WTC). This theory, originally developed by McCroskey and Richmond (1987), was subsequently modified by MacIntyre et al. (1998). It explains why some individuals are more willing than others to use their second (i.e., non-native) language in specific circumstances. This theory has been adapted to the health context (Baker & Watson, 2015) and is discussed later in this chapter. Other important theories of intergroup communication that have been researched in the health domain include the linguistic category model (LCM: Semin & Fiedler, 1991) and the theory of linguistic intergroup bias (LIB: Maass et al., 1989). All of these intergroup theories of communication serve to expand our understanding of health communication and work alongside one another to explain and predict communication behaviour. The following research demonstrates the value of an intergroup lens in the health domain.

Recent and Ongoing Intergroup Research into Doctor and Patient Communication

Over the past decade, Dr Susan Baker and I have expanded on earlier CAT findings concerning doctor and patient interactions. Baker adopted MacIntyre et al.'s (1998) theory of willingness to communicate (WTC) in a second language (Baker & MacIntyre, 2003) and extended it to the health sector. WTC in a language that is not the person's native language but rather a second language is very context specific. Macintyre argued that individuals who are trying to speak in a second language often feel inhibited among native speakers. He further argued that because they aren't native speakers, they will see themselves as outgroup members and so won't feel competent to speak in the second language.

Baker took this concept of second language group membership and adapted it to a health context (Baker, 2006). Knowing that individuals vary in the extent to which they are willing to communicate with doctors, she hypothesised that what influences their willingness to communicate will depend on both their confidence and their competence to interact lucidly with a doctor. Baker and Watson (2015) found that patients' own perceived level of health communication competence was the best predictor of their WTC. They also established that patients' reports of positive and negative experiences in consultations were correlated with their perceptions of the doctors' communication strategies. Baker et al. (2021) later established that their perceptions of how much they participated in consultations were positively correlated specifically with their perception of the particular doctor's level of emotional expression. In their study, patients described what made consultations with doctors satisfying or dissatisfying. Unsurprisingly, patients wanted time to tell their story. They reported needing to feel psychologically comfortable in the doctor's presence and wanted the doctor to listen to and respect what they said.

In another study, Baker and Watson (2020) investigated whether patients used health information on the internet to assist them with doctor-patient consultations. Three hundred and seventy participants from Australia and Canada completed a survey that included their rating of WTC in a health context, together with their rating of use and trust of the internet. Findings suggested that patients could recognise some websites as not trustworthy and could also discriminate between health information websites. Importantly, though, the study showed that patients with a high WTC were more likely to seek information before a consultation, so they could prepare themselves for their session. The information they gleaned from the internet allowed them to ask questions and actively participate in their consultation. By contrast, those participants with a low WTC score were more likely to use the internet after a consultation in order to make sense of what the doctor had told them. This second group also used the internet as a means of obtaining information in order to avoid visiting the doctor in the first place.

The foregoing studies by Susan Baker and myself are ongoing, but the initial message suggests that a patient's level of participation is associated with the emotional expression strategies used by the doctor. Alongside this, and what requires still more attention, is a patient's WTC with their doctor. Patients with low WTC may benefit from a doctor who is able to display attentive listening, a caring attitude, and an ability to take into account their specific concerns. In other words, patients are different, and ultimately their differences can impact the actual doctor-patient interaction. These studies again highlight the interplay between interpersonal and intergroup dynamics. By drawing on WTC in a health context, they have demonstrated how some patients may feel unwilling to talk to their doctor because they don't feel they have either the competence or the confidence to actively participate in a consultation. Using CAT, the studies have suggested that doctors can actively engage the strategies of emotional expression and discourse management in order to encourage participation from those patients with low WTC in health settings.

Up to this point, the focus has been on the medical practitioner. It's now time to review research conducted with health professionals other than doctors in order to discover the extent to which intergroup dynamics are in evidence there.

The Application of CAT: Patients and Various Health Professionals

Researchers who embrace an intergroup perspective have examined patient interactions other than those solely with doctors. For example, Bourhis et al. (1989) used CAT to discover the extent to which nurses and doctors used everyday language versus medical language when they conversed with the hospital patients. Their findings showed that nurses converged to medical language when speaking with doctors and to everyday language when speaking with patients. Nurses who converged towards the patients' language were seen by them as the communication brokers, mediating between the doctors and themselves. Doctors did not converge to everyday language when speaking with patients, which was problematic for patients because using everyday language for them led to better understanding. This early study was one of the first CAT studies to examine intergroup dynamics in a hospital context, and to explain differences in speech registers [2] (i.e., in how individuals modify their speech) between nurses, doctors and patients. Two factors emerged from Bourhis et al.'s study that are important features of communication.

The first factor was that the way an individual perceives they are speaking may not be corroborated when conversations are objectively observed by others. Doctors, in this study, reported that they employed a high use of everyday language with patients. By contrast, nurses and patients reported that doctors actually used low levels of everyday language. A more recent study by Zimmermann and Jucks (2018) showed the importance for experts to gauge accurately the comprehension competence of the receivers of their message. In their study, experts provided nutritional advice to other experts. and to laypersons. The experts provided this information at an appropriate technical level when presenting to experts, and then used everyday language to laypersons. They also reversed this manipulation, providing information using technical terms to the laypersons and everyday language to the experts. Their study demonstrated that when experts gave advice that was unsuited to the recipients' comprehension level, it was viewed as non-accommodative and reduced the recipients' levels of trust and credibility. This finding has serious implications for ensuring that doctors are trusted and that treatment plans are understood and followed by patients.

The second factor that emerged from the study was the importance of group membership in the hospital context. They demonstrated that group memberships (e.g., doctors, nurses and patients) are highly salient and influence how a member of one group believes they should communicate with a member of another group. Their study showed that individuals are often unaware of how their communication choices may fail to meet the comprehension needs of their speech partner. CAT clearly indicates why individuals are misunderstood and provides strategies to make health professionals and their patients better communicators. CAT emphasises that a speaker should avoid making any preliminary assumptions

---

2 "Register: A variety of language related to the social context. A speaker may vary their vocabulary, tone and level of formality to reflect the audience and purpose within a situation".

about their interactant. It is understandable that it happens, but in health consultations, assumptions must be made conscious and be tested by the speakers.

This study by Bourhis et al. (1989) suggests that compared with doctors, nurses may be more effective communicators with patients in a hospital context because they are better able to address the patients' comprehension needs (interpretability). This finding raises the question of whether patients find it easier to talk about their health concerns with nurses rather than doctors. If patients do find nurses more accessible to their needs, it may be because nurses necessarily spend more time with patients in a ward than do doctors. Greater familiarity with their patients may mean that many topics beyond treatment and illness are discussed, so establishing a rapport between them. Nurses may be more approachable than doctors, and their lower status in the hospital system could be one reason for this. These findings were mirrored more recently by Clayton et al. (2021), who reiterated that nurses are trained in communicating over a wide range of topics with patients and have the most interaction with them.

Jones et al. (2018) examined nurse interactions in a neonatal unit, focusing on the importance of emotional expression as a CAT strategy. They noted that nurses provided lower levels of emotional expression to adolescent mothers than to mothers in the more typical childbearing age group. Nurses reported having less empathy with the younger mothers, even though they required at least as much emotional support as the older women. This need for such emotional support was also demonstrated by Sheeran et al. (2013), who found that adolescent mothers described nurses as unsupportive, using inappropriate interpersonal control that led to them feeling unempowered and marginalised.

Importantly, the communication strategies applied by nurses in these two studies demonstrate how robustly CAT is able to identify which communication strategies and associated specific behaviours lead to evaluations of ineffective versus effective interaction. The study by Jones et al. (2018) focused on nurses' reports, whereas the Sheeran et al. study concentrated on the mothers' reports. The findings from both studies confirm that the strategies identified by CAT are insightful into both the way interaction unfolds and the effects of communication behaviours on each speech partner. Qualitative research by Jones et al. (2015) investigated both nurses' and parents' perceptions of communication in a pre-term babies' nursery. Using semi-structured interviews, they found that while both groups concentrated on communication that equipped them for caring, nurses defined such enablement in different ways. Some nurses expected parents to do as they were instructed, while others encouraged the parents to be independent. These different nurse expectations led to difficulties and conflict for the parents. Some of the nurse participants also stereotyped the parents into specific categories. If nurses categorised parents as too young, or drug dependent, or from particular ethnic and cultural groups, communication could be compromised. Some parents spoke about being made to feel "stupid" and "incompetent", while one mother felt she was discriminated against by the nurses because she was older with a younger partner (Jones et al., 2015, p. 6).

Another finding from their study highlighted how hospital policy can cause conflict when applied inconsistently. This sometimes occurred because staff didn't know the specific hospital policy or simply chose to ignore it. At other times, it seemed nurses viewed policy as intransigent. Parents found this confusing and upsetting. The parents' experience of such inconsistency reflects the fact that the hospital system itself is yet another factor that drives the way communication proceeds, and this again can be a cause of miscommunication. The aspect of hospital systems is further explored in Chapter 6. Interestingly, the nurses interviewed in the Jones et al. study did not appreciate how impactful were their communication interactions with parents. Parents, on the other hand, reported needing reassurance and supportive communication from nurses. All of these findings demonstrate intergroup dynamics in the way they highlight the social roles of the interactants and the constraints on how communication unfolds.

Venning and colleagues (2000) discussed the role of nurses qualified as nurse practitioners in primary care, finding that patients reported higher satisfaction levels with them than with doctors. A systematic review in 2002 corroborated this conclusion (Horrocks et al., 2002). A more recent review by Torrens et al. (2020) examined barriers and facilitators affecting the employment of nurse practitioners. It provided a balanced discussion of existing barriers, including those affecting teams and the degree of acceptance from doctors and other health professionals of the nurse practitioner's role. From an intergroup perspective, this requires more in-depth investigation. As will be shown in Chapter 4, resistance to nurse specialisation can be toxic. In some cases, patients may gain a better understanding of their condition by accepting the nurse as a communication broker between themselves and doctors. Formally adopting such a relationship within a system could promote greater patient adherence to treatment, resulting in better patient outcomes. An LSP approach would expand understanding of these issues and certainly be worth future application.

In the late 1990s, research by Watson and Gallois (1998, 1999) explored how accommodative and non-accommodative communication strategies were associated with patient satisfaction and willingness to adhere to treatment. They examined how patients perceived their interactions with a range of health providers: doctors, nurses and other health professionals. Their findings highlighted the multifaceted nature of communication strategies, as well as the intergroup nature of patient and provider interactions. More specifically, the studies revealed that while patients were accepting of the health professionals' authority as experts, they also wanted to exert some level of control during the consultation. For example, when patients perceived that health professionals were directive in consultations to ensure appropriate treatment, but also perceived that they were acknowledged as individuals with specific needs, they gave high satisfaction ratings. Unsatisfactory consultations occurred when health professionals took sole charge and didn't give patients the opportunity to express their own opinions. Relatedly, when health professionals used accommodative discourse management, patients perceived they were able to share the floor and felt listened to. It was actually from this health communication research that the emotional expression communication strategy was developed.

A key finding was that patients wanted health professionals to show appropriate concern and reassurance (Watson & Gallois, 1998, 1999). Emotional expression was one of the strongest predictors of patient satisfaction and positive evaluation of the healthcare consultation. In contrast, interpretability was not a predictor of satisfactory consultations, indicating that patients do not use this strategy to judge health providers as poor communicators. What matters to patients is that the health professional has ensured they are allowed to engage in the consultation, ask questions, and feel emotionally supported. This was confirmed in the previously described studies by Baker and colleagues (Baker & Watson, 2015; Baker et al., 2021). The balance between seeing a patient as an individual (high interpersonal salience) and viewing the patient only as a patient with health issues (high intergroup salience) appears to be critical. These findings by Watson and Gallois applied to all types of health professionals; professions were not analysed separately.

What insights can we derive by applying an LSP perspective to the intergroup dynamics within an interaction? Certainly, a person's social and cultural identities often play an important role in how they see interactants and how interactants see them. At any given moment, such encounters are driven by the rules and cultural expectations associated with each salient group identity. As I've indicated earlier, health interactions are a very specific type of encounter; being the patient or the treating health professional influences the progress of the communication process. We saw above how nurses in the neonatal intensive care unit treated young mothers differently and with less respect than they did older mothers. It is noteworthy that a growing number of practising health professionals have adopted an intergroup approach to analyse health interactions (e.g., Barlow et al., 2024; Chevalier et al., 2017; Hewett et al., 2009). This is important because it demonstrates that health providers identify and recognise the influence of the intergroup environment. These three last-named researchers provide their own perspectives in the final chapter.

Moving the Focus to Pharmacists

For her doctoral thesis, Bernadette Chevalier, a practising pharmacist, invoked CAT to explore communication effectiveness between hospital pharmacists and patients during medication counselling. Medication counselling takes place when a hospital inpatient is discharged and is provided with information about their drug-taking regimen. A number of interesting findings emerged, reflecting earlier findings in doctor–patient interactions. In one of her studies, pharmacists stated their goals for patient interaction. They reported wanting to build patient rapport, to ensure that their patients felt empowered and to improve patients' experience in the consultation as well as their health and safety (Chevalier et al., 2016).

However, a further study by Chevalier et al. (2017) showed that while pharmacists employed all five CAT strategies (see Chapter 2 of this book), they did not always provide a clear agenda for the medication counselling sessions, nor did they use open-ended questions or invite patient input. One reason given by the pharmacists for this lack of structure and reduced patient engagement was time pressures within the hospital system, another sign that hospitals do not promote a climate for effective communication. Chevalier and colleagues also found that the pharmacists' self-rating of their use of the communication strategies did not always match that of an outside observer (a pharmacist) of the patient and pharmacist consultations. Specifically, pharmacists tended to rate themselves more highly on demonstrating effective emotional expression and discourse management, but gave themselves lower ratings on interpretability and interpersonal control.

Once again, such findings demonstrate the way that CAT reveals the lack of concordance between how an individual believes they are behaving and how they are observed to behave. In Chapter 7, I discuss software used by Chevalier and colleagues that enabled pharmacists to measure precisely their communication behaviours with patients (Chevalier et al., 2018). Chevalier et al.'s work also shows how patients and pharmacists have similar goals for their interaction, resulting in complementary behaviours. For example, pharmacists wanted patients to be confident about their ability to organise medication intake. Patients shared this goal. To this end, patients tended to focus on medication details provided by the pharmacist and on the pharmacist's personal manner. Pharmacists focused on ensuring the patient understood the information through their active participation. However, many interactions with outgoing patients were rushed due to a lack of sufficient time. We should also bear in mind that a newly discharged patient may be at the mercy of a transport system to take them home and may be anxious simply to leave the hospital. These concerns about organising homeward travel can be a serious and distracting concern for patients, and can make them less receptive and attentive to information provided by the pharmacist.

Futile Care

This last topic is highly sensitive but provides valuable insights into how healthcare is negotiated in the hospital context. Gallois et al. (2015) conducted research into how health professionals, patients and other relevant carers negotiate decisions about end-of-life treatment. Such treatment, referred to as "futile care", does not benefit the patient and indeed may actually cause suffering. Gallois and colleagues (2015) noted that the communication processes for end-of-life treatment are not well researched. They invoked the Linguistic Category Model (LCM) developed by Gun Semin and Klaus Fiedler (1992). The LCM complements CAT by revealing that we tend to use positive and enduring terms to describe our ingroups but more negative and enduring terms when describing an outgroup. By "enduring" I mean not a solitary or one-off behaviour, but one that is repeated; for example, I might say that my ingroup is friendly but that my outgroup is hostile. These will be continuing perceptions. Gallois and colleagues emphasised that the recognition of an intergroup component in what at first sight appears to be only an interpersonal situation expands our perspective and understanding of how communication and related behaviour play out. While there is most definitely an interpersonal dimension to discussing end-of-life care, it often occurs within the health context, which is an established intergroup domain (see Barlow et al., 2024; Setchell et al., 2015; Watson et al., 2016).

Gallois et al. (2015) demonstrated the presence of group identity salience in their interviews with 96 medical doctors. These doctors used language demonstrating that they held differing opinions on their ingroup's (i.e., same health specialty and seniority) end-of-life care compared to their outgroups (i.e., different health specialties or seniority levels). When doctors described the futile care that they and their ingroup colleagues might have provided, they spoke of giving family or patients more time to come to terms with end-of-life. They spoke of considering the pros and cons of continuing treatment and, provided it benefited the patient and family and did not incur excessive financial cost to the community, whether it was appropriate. As Gallois et al. (2015) predicted, doctors employed positive enduring terms in their assessments of their own and their ingroup's choice of futile care. When they spoke of using futile care, it was often because they wanted to respect the wishes of the patient or the family. Gallois et al. pointed out that, in this instance, the patient and family are the outgroup driving the use of extended treatment. A doctor exonerated themself by saying "I will always respect the competent patient's wishes, I won't go against them" (Gallois et al., 2015, p. 664). One junior doctor stated that the senior doctor (the consultant) had recommended a course of treatment which they believed futile. Nevertheless, the prescribed medication was administered, but by the less painful of alternative methods. Even though the junior doctor considered the treatment futile and not appropriate, it was important both to obey the consultant and to reduce the patient's discomfort as much as possible.

In contrast, doctors reported experiencing conflict with their outgroup colleagues with respect to futile care. They used enduring negative language to describe the outgroup members' reasoning for providing futile care. One doctor commented on outgroup doctors and their decision to continue treatment as follows: "Worst offenders are the haematology and oncology people who are still giving chemotherapy to people, $20,000 a month when they're riddled with tumours basically everywhere. I think it's a criminal waste of money personally" (Gallois et al., 2015, p. 667). Junior doctors are obliged to acquiesce to the senior doctor. The junior doctor may adapt the recommended treatment by administering it in ways they see as more appropriate. This can be problematic for their patient if the two doctors do not fully agree on the precise care procedures.

Spoken and Written Communication are Both Important

Health communication is varied and complex. Health communication researchers have paid greater attention to patient and physician interactions at the expense of those between patients and other health professionals. It is abundantly clear that the profession of the health provider can influence the communication behaviours of the patient. This is an important finding. It should be utilised to discover the reasons for behavioural differences and to investigate what can be done to enhance or reduce them. The different communication styles of doctors and patients go beyond spoken communication. A glance at the notes written on an inpatient's medical record, for example, can reveal different approaches to patient care. Leonard et al. (2004) observed the difference between doctors and nurses in their writing up of patient medical records. They noted that nurses tended to write a highly descriptive narrative about the patient, covering their day-to-day health activities, while doctors did not. Rather, the doctors' input to medical patient records was much more succinct and might comprise only a few words and diagrams. Doctors often apply the acronym SOAP to help them formulate a care plan: Subjective, Objective, Assessment, Plan. This refers to the doctor's subjective and objective observations, their subsequent assessment of what that means, and how it will inform their plan for treatment. Foronda et al. (2016) examined instances of miscommunication between nurses and physicians. A fundamental cause was that the two professions are trained with very different approaches to patient care, and this is reflected in their different styles of communication. Both approaches are correct, and both matter, but the differences between them speak volumes about how nurses and doctors manage and focus on patient care. These points are taken up in the next chapter.

During my own research, nurses have said to me that they are there to care for the patients. They are often the first to recognise when family and friends should be called. Doctors, they said, often want to continue with more treatment. The patient's connection with their nurse and with their doctor illustrates two very different approaches to patient care.

Review

What are the takeaway messages from this chapter? There are so many other areas that this chapter could have covered, e.g., aged care facilities, or carers dealing with dementia or schizophrenia. All these contexts are important and complex, and the intergroup and interpersonal salience in any one of these contexts and encounters will most likely vary. But I hope the message is clear. The organisational system within which healthcare exists, the professional roles and identities of the health providers, and, in varying degrees, the patient's identity as they adhere to or resist care, all set up an intergroup dynamic. It is an "us" and "them" if you will. It is imperative that the intergroup dynamic be recognised because it informs how interactions proceed. And it is the actions that arise from those interactions that influence patient care and wellbeing.

Some Personal Review Points

This chapter has covered the complex connections that exist between health professionals and their patients. Our doctor at the beginning of the chapter spoke about building close relationships with their patients and how seeing each person as an individual is so important.

- What are your experiences of forming relationships with patients?
- How much do you consider the individual characteristics of a patient in a consultation?

- Does focusing on the patient as a unique person with likes and dislikes make the consultation more effective for you? If yes, why? If no, why not?

In the next chapter, the focus moves away from patients and their health providers to that of health professionals engaging with other health professionals in order to negotiate and safely manage patient care.

Communication Between Health Professionals from Different Disciplines

What does it mean to work collaboratively with health professionals from different disciplines? In this recorded extract, a senior social worker from a metropolitan hospital in Queensland, Australia, gives their opinion about working in multidisciplinary teams:

Look – it's your multidisciplinary communication and doing that on a regular basis. We changed from a system where we would meet twice a week for a couple of hours with the medical doctors and allied health and nursing staff on a ward. We found that things were kind of waiting for these meetings, so they might be on a Wednesday and a Thursday. Something may happen on a Monday, but we'll say let's wait until the meeting on Wednesday – there is almost two days of nothing happening for the patient. So, we developed a daily – what they call rapid rounds – where you sit down – the whole treating team – sits down and goes through every single patient, every single day. Now that's got its own kind of problems around, perhaps not getting the detail and focusing on some things and not on other things. But in terms of the communication between the disciplines, there is that regular feedback, there's that regular update, and that regular opportunity for everyone to have their input with everyone hearing the same story. A doctor might say they want to go – um, "oh we want to discharge them today" but the physio will go, "well no, they're not safe, they still need one person assist", the occupational therapist might go, "well they have cognitive issues which we need to assess further", and the social worker might go, "well there is carer stress". Perhaps in the past that would have taken a few days to have that conversation; this can happen every day. And we can get referrals earlier as opposed to waiting a couple of days. When they come in, we're meeting at the next morning, and we are knowing at 8 o'clock the next morning about potential referrals so we can get on to them quicker.

This shows quite clearly how teamwork can be effective when each health provider is given an opportunity to offer their opinion. It's a positive example of effective communication, and it demonstrates how staff well-being is enhanced when teams collaborate.

In this chapter, I shall look closely at how health professionals manage patient care when several become involved in a treatment plan, and I'll explain how such care can occur collaboratively or independently across a number of different contexts. I'll examine how research by academics has tried to improve communication between different health professionals, despite paying minimal attention to the dynamics of intergroup communication. And finally, I'll show that the professional identities of different health providers are often directly responsible for unsatisfactory communication in discussions about patient care management. Greater awareness of this last situation would assist in making communication far more transparent and collaborative than is currently the case.

As in the previous chapter, the problems discussed here are not new; they are recurring issues in healthcare. What is new is the application of an LSP approach to examine them. By advocating LSP, I don't imply that other perspectives aren't also valuable; we should be expanding upon the research perspectives that have already been used. An LSP approach shows why an intergroup focus is needed for investigation. I'll be examining just a representative sample of situations in which health professionals talk to each other about patient care. Nowadays, discussions between different health professionals are a normal and regular occurrence. They may be from the same or different professions, and they will often vary in seniority, but in each case my focus will be on how well they negotiate and share knowledge regarding a patient's treatment plan, because such negotiation is vital to ensure quality treatment outcomes.

Shared Patient Care

Historically, it was the doctor who took charge of a patient and oversaw their care, but now shared patient care is an everyday event. One of the simplest examples is that of a GP wanting more information about a patient's current health status. The GP may order a blood test, which the patient will then have taken via pathology. The system of returning a blood test report to the GP will require collaboration with the pathologist, and the results will assist the GP in deciding the next step in the patient's care. This might be to do nothing if the results are good, to decide on a course of medication to treat a condition identified by the results, or to refer the patient to a specialist for further consultation. Should the third option be taken, then the GP will, at some later point, receive a report from the specialist on the patient's health status. This report may leave the patient in the complete care of the GP, or it may result in the specialist taking over care or even referring the patient to other specialists for further treatment. It does not take long for many health professionals to become involved in one patient's care. This shared care, when it works well, is often seamless and will be familiar to many of us.

However, medical and technological advances have resulted in patients now living with sometimes complex conditions. Patients with comorbidities often need treatment from a range of disciplines, thus requiring a number of specialist doctors to treat particular aspects of their illness. Previously, such multiple care was not possible; the comorbidities would almost inevitably have shortened patients' lives. Patients suffering from diabetes, for example, are now normally seen by a number of different health providers including their GP, an endocrinologist and a dietitian. If the diabetes causes further health problems, care may extend to others such as an ophthalmologist or cardiologist. Such shared patient care requires health providers and specialists to work in teams and communicate effectively with each other to determine the right treatment plan. Knowing what medications each doctor has prescribed is vital; if this information isn't shared, it can lead to contraindications where a mixture of drugs causes negative reactions. Communication between professions can so easily become fragmented, often leading to problems with patient care.

A person admitted as a hospital inpatient will also experience shared care. They will see numerous health professionals who will independently doubtless ask the patient many of the same as well as different questions. Answering the same questions repeatedly can make an already ill patient anxious and can be exhausting for them. A small study conducted by Whitt et al. (2007) confirmed that patients see a large number and a wide range of health providers while in hospital. Their study included only health professionals who recorded their visit in the patient's medical record, so the actual number of professionals consulting with the patient could be even larger. Whitt and colleagues emphasised the need for ensuring effective communication, not only between the health professionals but also between health professionals and their patients. Whitt et al. (2007) focused on the organisational structure of hospitals, identifying the complex systems within which health professionals work as a potentially serious hindrance to effective communication.

Why would communication not be effective between different health professionals? I've touched on this when discussing the strong hierarchical and power status differentials that exist between the different healthcare professions (see Chapter 2). Junior doctors may not check any misunderstanding when interacting with a senior consultant for fear of appearing incompetent. Hewett et al. (2009)

investigated communication between hospital doctors and its impact on the quality of patient care. They interviewed 45 doctors and invoked SIT and CAT to understand how professional identity and intergroup relationships are expressed when doctors specialising in different medical disciplines interact with each other.

Hewett and colleagues investigated the extent to which accommodative and non-accommodative CAT strategies were evident during communication. The represented specialties comprised Internal Medicine, Gastroenterology and Hepatology, General Surgery, Anaesthesia and Perioperative Medicine, Intensive Care Medicine and Medical Administration. The doctors were all involved in the care of patients who presented at the Department of Emergency with an upper gastrointestinal bleed. This condition can be life-threatening. Hewett et al. (2009) found that all doctors viewed their own specialty as highly salient, something plainly evident from their indiscriminate referral to other doctors as belonging to specific groups by familiarly shortening them, e.g., gastroenterologists as "gastros" and Department of Emergency Medicine as "DEM" (p. 1736). Such labelling spotlighted how difficult it can be to collaborate, one doctor even describing how a "turf war" existed between the different specialties (p. 1736).

This study identified clear areas of conflict, one being the administration policies. For example, one such policy stated that the doctor responsible for admitting the patient effectively owned that patient and was ultimately responsible for their treatment. Other specialties were present only to consult. The following two quotations from doctors involved make this point clear. A General Medicine specialist spoke about patient ownership: "Everybody's got a different version of what's a surgical patient and what's a medical patient and the grey area is fought out, patient by patient, in Emergency every day. And the surgeons will say, no it's not a surgical patient .... they lose their ownership of the problem and they're not directly responsible, so they don't feel any need to visit every day and see that patient" (Hewett et al., 2009, p. 1736). A DEM registrar made the point that: "There are definitely situations where, if there are multiple teams involved in their ongoing management, no one wants to buy-in to be the primary responsible person .... and there's disagreements about who's going to be primarily responsible" (1736–1737).

Both quotations reveal a conflictual environment for patient care. Hewett and colleagues (2009) analysed the presence of accommodative and non-accommodative stances. When senior doctors worked with other senior doctors, they tended to communicate by focusing on their interpersonal identity rather than their department identity. This, they reported, led to communication at a senior level working well. However, counter-accommodation was described by some senior doctors when they spoke to more junior doctors. The following excerpt illustrates a senior gastroenterology consultant putting pressure on an anaesthetic registrar (who is more junior) to ensure early access to a procedure for a patient. The consultant stated:

"But I think that when problems arise the consultant has to sort it out. My first port of call always is to ring the registrar who's been involved with my registrar and make it very clear and to put pressure on them. And say: 'What is going on? What is the delay? What are you doing about it?' And put big pressure on them. And then, if that's not going well, I'd say: 'Who's your consultant? Who's on tonight?' 'Bill Smith'. 'Well, is Dr Smith here?' 'No, he's at home'. 'Right. Well, perhaps I need to speak to Dr Smith because, you need to'. And then usually, they fold. Because, you see, these things don't worry me. I mean, no one likes an argument, and I find it unpleasant. But, you see, I don't feel any threat from this place. I have an awful lot of skills and some skills that no one else has. I'd be better to have the afternoon off and catch up on paperwork or have dinner with my family" (Hewett et al., 2009, p. 1737).

A final focus of Hewett et al.'s study was the impact on the quality of patient care, as the following excerpt demonstrates. (Fortunately, the patient involved was eventually treated because the Department of Emergency Medicine specialist moved the problem to the Director of Gastroenterology, who agreed on the procedure.)

"I was taking over from someone and they said, 'Oh, this bloke here, he's got a foreign body impacted in his oesophagus', which is a relative emergency. 'But they're not going to scope him until they've got a bed.' I said, 'You're kidding.' 'No, no, that's right. Look, they've written it in the chart.' The gastroenterology registrar had actually written, 'Not to come up for scope until bed available.' … And, once again, in an attempt to put us over the barrel and say, 'Look, if you can take them back, we'll take them and scope them now.' 'No, I'm sorry, that's your decision. This patient needs a scope. Take it up with the Med Super.' See, that's just outrageous! This patient needs to have something done. You have the capacity to do it right now. What do you think your ass is going to look like if something bad happens – if that guy ruptures his oesophagus because, 'Oh, there's no bed and we can't look after him in recovery after he has his scope.' You're not going to have a leg to stand on." (Hewett et al., 2009 p. 1738).

We can see a description of a highly conflictual event with clear hostilities at play. This study by Hewett et al. (2009) concluded that doctors were working in highly stressful situations that regularly led to intergroup conflict and counter-accommodative interactions. The authors suggested that multiple ownership of a patient would assist this volatile climate and might encourage more accommodative interpersonal interactions. I've concentrated on this study because it explains quite neatly the issues that different specialties can face when managing a patient's admission to the hospital. However, once a patient is admitted, shared care continues.

Clinical Handovers

Another form of shared care is the clinical handover. This can take many forms. It includes, but is not limited to, shift-to-shift handover where the outgoing shift transfers patient information to the incoming shift. Shift handover can occur between nurses only or with both doctors and nurses present. Another form of handover is the case conference, where a number of health professionals come together to discuss the care of patients on a particular ward or unit. There are also handovers between hospital wards or units when, for example, a patient is transferred from the emergency department to a hospital ward, or post-operative handovers when a patient comes back from the operating theatre into recovery and then back to the ward. Aside from these handover variations, of which there are many, there are also informal discussions between doctors about a patient's care, and out-of-hours phone calls to an on-call physician. This last usually occurs if a patient is judged by a nurse or junior doctor on duty to be deteriorating. Handover has been an important research area for many health scholars for more than two decades (Abraham et al., 2014). The broad scope of clinical handover is one reason so much effort and time have been spent on trying to improve the process. There is, however, one universally agreed fact about handover: it is the weak link in the chain of patient care (Koch et al., 2014; Robertson et al., 2014). Vital patient information can be missed and so not communicated, or when it is communicated, it can be misunderstood by the receiver of the handover with sometimes disastrous results. Many resources and interventions have been designed to improve this "weak link". But the problem still remains.

One study has explored how different hospital health professionals perceived issues with handover (Watson et al., 2014). Using a software mining tool called Leximancer, the study examined the similarities and differences existing between the perceptions of health professionals when each described barriers to effective handover (see Chapter 7 for a discussion of Leximancer). Findings revealed that all health professionals saw managing their time as an issue that affected them personally. They all spoke of time management, time pressures, and difficulties around coordinating different handovers. However, each profession described their problem with time differently. Nurses emphasised the role of time in relation to the quality of the information transmitted at the handover, some suggesting time constraints be put on nurse handovers in order to reduce the inclusion of unnecessary information. Doctors stressed the importance of presenting information in a clear format. The introduction of a template for handover content was seen by them as a way to ensure structured patient information, but they also noted that because they were so busy, there was actually insufficient time to complete the template.

The central time issue for allied health professionals was that they worked across many hospital wards, making it often impossible to attend the handovers of all the patients for whom they were responsible. They said there were just too many wards and that they could not physically get to them all. What mattered to them was seeking out the correct person who could explain the handover decisions that had been made during their working day. A second separate analysis conducted in this study revealed that each profession also focused on separate aspects of handover. Nurses discussed the downsides of taped handovers rather than live ones. This style of handover, unique to nurses, has now become less common because of safety concerns (Australian Commission on Safety and Quality in Health Care, 2012). Doctors commented that they found it difficult to organise seeing all the registrars to discuss details about patients admitted to the hospital. They emphasised that the medical staff needed to be able to access their colleagues at times other than at handover, and that not being able to do so was problematic for their patient care management. In contrast, the allied health professionals were more concerned with future plans for the patients rather than their immediate care needs.

This study nicely illustrates how health providers focus on different aspects of patient care and face different challenges as they deal with attending handovers. Watson et al. (2014) also observed the frustration of health professionals because they did not have the authority to alter the organisational structures and policies that determined handover timing and procedure. For example, doctors were keen for nurses to attend the morning handover but realised this wasn't always possible because it took place at the same time as the nurses were at their busiest on the wards, attending to their patients' daily assisted living needs.

Teamwork and its Associated Problems

Aside from handover, a team of diverse health professionals may need to work together on one patient's care. Victims of cerebrovascular accidents, for example, routinely have a group of health professionals working on their rehabilitation. Their treatment plan will be decided by the particular group of health disciplines responsible for its coordination. Such a team is often called a multidisciplinary team because it works collaboratively in its decision-making: the whole team is actively involved. Although the terms multidisciplinary team and interdisciplinary team are often used interchangeably, the former differs fundamentally by its emphasis on collaborative knowledge sharing about the patient between its separate members. The members of an interdisciplinary team, on the other hand, often work independently of each other and so constitute a team in name only. Each professional will manage the patient's care independently without collaborative consultation. Patient notes may be available to all concerned, but shared decision-making about a collaborative treatment plan does not occur. In this situation, there is a danger that one or more of the health providers caring for the patient will be unaware of the treatment plans of the other practitioners or related medical prescriptions. If patient notes are not regularly checked by all health providers, problems can arise with a consequent detrimental effect on patient care.

Lorelei Lingard is a world-renowned scholar who sees medical discourse as a social activity shaped by the health provider's professional identity. Although Lingard does not invoke social identity theory or CAT per se, her findings complement these theories. She has observed that health professionals working independently can be extremely competent. However, when two or more health professionals form a team, although they can sometimes still retain their competence and work well together, more often than not they become collectively incompetent and regrettably do not work well together. Why is this? There is no one answer, but rather a number of circumstances that, taken together, have militated against good teamwork between health professionals. There are always exceptions, but for the most part, health providers do not work well when they come together to exchange information and co-manage patient care.

Lingard offers some interesting insights into this complex problem. Her chapter in a book she edited with Brian Hodges focuses on the nature of health professional competence (Lingard, 2012). Here she elaborates on her own theoretical perspective. (I can strongly recommend it as an excellent read.) With respect to health professionals and teamwork, she makes the following observations. Medical education at the university focuses on individual learning; students are assessed on their competency as individuals. An example of this is the all-important objective structured clinical examination (OSCE) in which medical students are tested individually on their ability to diagnose and treat standardised patients. In addition, Lingard notes that practitioners bill their patients individually. She observes that assessing a medical practitioner as competent implies that they will be competent across the different and varying contexts of their work. But in reality, it is by no means the case that someone who interacts well with one specific health profession is thereby able to work well with other professions.

The individual focus of training does not allow for a thorough assessment of collaboration with others. A person in any profession may differ in the extent to which they are a team player. I have worked with many academics, and I know that their recognised high level of expert knowledge may not translate into an ability to work with others in a team, e.g., to collaborate on a research project. It does not necessarily come naturally to them, and there may be other reasons why collaboration does not occur.

Lingard's final point concerning competency is that in the medical field (as elsewhere), the health provider must be continually upskilling so as to ensure that their knowledge remains current. If this does not occur, then the health provider's level of competency will be found wanting. Lingard makes the insightful comment that being a qualified medical practitioner with many years of experience paradoxically may mean they are not as competent or up to date as those more recently trained. Time, in this instance, regardless of accrued experience, reduces competency levels. These perceptions of what it means to be competent reflect the focus on the individual and how competency is measured. She therefore proposes that being competent needs to include being able to work collaboratively in teams and, to this end, highlights the concept of collective competency: the competency of the team as a whole to work as a cohesive unit. In sum, she argues that medical practitioners need to be given opportunities throughout their careers to demonstrate their continuing competence across different situations and with different teams.

Relatedly, the term silo mentality has been used in medicine to describe how health professionals work. In general, they are not taught to discuss or debate their patients' care with other disciplines. Physicians are taught from the beginning of their careers that they are the ones in charge of patient care and that the responsibility for a patient's outcome rests with them. From both Lingard's understanding of healthcare interactions and from an intergroup perspective, current approaches to teaching are clearly unhelpful and potentially dangerous for the patient with multiple needs from several professions.

Interprofessional Practice

The pervasive intergroup environment in hospitals is, as already explained, due to the power differentials between professions, the resultant hierarchical structure of the organisation, and the importance that individuals attach to their professional identity. A health provider's profession defines who they are in the organisational culture, situates them within the hierarchy, and provides them with a sense of belonging. A key issue here is that those working within the hospital system do not always recognise how that system influences their judgement and subsequent communication behaviour. This was recognised by Coupland et al. (1991) who observed that "miscommunication resides in group and cultural phenomena" (p. 13). In other words, learned communication behaviours are so deeply entrenched in the organisational culture that those within it do not see the problem or, if they do, feel that nothing can be changed because that is how the culture operates.

Importantly, it is not just the health professions that fall into the silo trap. Hospital staff working in human and financial resources, as well as policy and administrative staff, are all situated somewhere in the system, communicating within their own silos. My own research has often revealed how practitioners see management and administration as the enemy who don't understand what frontline staff need in order to provide quality patient care. They simply impose budgetary constraints that lead to longer working hours for health providers and fewer staff to care for patients. We know that health systems across the globe are at breaking point. Industrial action for these very reasons was threatened in the UK during the summer of 2024. Employee stress, burnout and related staff shortages inevitably give rise to conflict. Administrators and policy makers are seen as outgroup members, often exacerbating a "them and us" mentality. It should not surprise us that the resulting high levels of intergroup conflict can adversely affect communication. While Coupland and colleagues' 1991 chapter is now over 30 years old, most regrettably their observation still holds true. The problem of individual competency and working *in silos* remains to be resolved.

In the 1980s, a concerted global effort was made to alter this silo mentality by encouraging health professionals from different disciplines to learn together (Anderson & Lennox, 2009). The World Health Organization produced the document *The Framework for Action on Interprofessional Education and Collaborative Practice*, a landmark in the new thinking on professional practice education (World Health Organization, 2010). For a comprehensive review of how interprofessional education (IPE) developed at the beginning of the twenty-first century, see Frenk et al. (2010). The basic principles of IPE were concerned with improving the skill sets of students undertaking health degrees (e.g., medicine, nursing and physical therapy), and equally their ability to share knowledge and negotiate patient care management. The rationale behind this new approach was the belief that if health professional undergraduates from different disciplines learned and worked together, an ethos of collaborative teamwork would emerge. This, in turn, it was argued, would lead to improved sharing and understanding of many medical terms that had previously not been universally used. However, the challenge was, and still is today, to carry over IPE at the undergraduate level to interprofessional practice (IPP) in the hospital environment. IPE learnings readily accepted by undergraduates must also be accepted by the hospital health professionals who work in a traditionally silo mentality. To date, no such transfer of practice from university to hospital has been achieved. The question we must ask is: Why not? Of course, there is no one answer; that would be simplistic, but applying an intergroup lens will help us unpack some of the issues that continue to exist.

Some hospitals have been aware of the poor communication existing between health professionals, and consequently have developed many training interventions in an attempt to reduce the problem. However, through their limitations, these interventions have, for the most part, failed. They have concentrated on the provision of training in communication competency skills, but this approach has assumed that miscommunication between individuals occurs simply because one or more have a skills deficit. A premise of what is termed intercultural communication competence (ICC) is that increasing knowledge about cultural norms will improve communication between individuals from different geographic cultures and so reduce or prevent miscommunication. This approach has proved useful within many contexts, but in a health context it is insufficient by itself to fully address the problem. See Chapter Five for a more detailed discussion.

Both health researchers and health practitioners have sought to solve the problem of miscommunication by treating interactions between health professionals as interpersonal encounters. The application of ICC by educators in a health context acknowledges that health professionals from different disciplines have different medical jargon and different cultures. It also recognises that they work *in silos*. Patients, too, are included in this approach, because just as health professionals have different cultural norms, so do patients. As noted by Teal and Street (2009), interactions between patients and health providers are intercultural encounters, so applying an ICC approach that highlights good communication skills is crucial to achieving their improvement.

So why, we must ask, have the many and various problems in communication not been eradicated from hospitals? There are at least two ICC issues which explain why communication is not always effective in healthcare. Firstly, the ICC approach, while insightful, does not consider each speaker's attitude towards their speech partner or the context of the conversation. As we've seen in earlier chapters, a person's attitude towards their interactant is an important driver of communication goals. A senior doctor, for example, may inform a junior doctor about a course of treatment for a patient. This will be a routine event for the senior doctor who will expect the junior to listen and follow instructions. They may assume the junior to be unfamiliar with certain advanced medical terms and so may deliberately use terms they believe are less technical. The junior doctor, new and relatively inexperienced, will almost certainly be extremely anxious to impress the senior doctor. Despite the senior doctor's best efforts to limit medical jargon, the junior may still not fully follow all the details of the required treatment. They will not, of course, wish to appear incompetent and so may well decide it better simply to nod and listen, and look up the unfamiliar details later (see Chapter 2 for details on communication strategies). It would be more sensible and appropriate for the junior to check understanding with the senior doctor immediately, but the cultural norms of the hospital hierarchy will militate against such behaviour. It's equally true that the senior doctor should check the junior's understanding. Sometimes this may occur, but often it may not, due to the embedded hierarchical culture. And even if the senior doctor does check understanding, it may again be the case that the junior will pretend to understand rather than admit ignorance or appear incompetent. The junior doctor will doubtless check another source as soon as possible, but there is now room for potentially serious error, as any delay will increase the risk of their misremembering or misinterpretation.

Secondly, the ICC approach assumes that the interactants in an encounter are working towards a positive and successful interaction for everyone concerned. However, if an individual has a negative attitude towards their speech partner, they may seek to make the conversation difficult. From an intergroup perspective, this is not uncommon. For a case in point, see the quote by the consultant in this chapter on page 43. Researchers in the health domain have demonstrated how one health professional sometimes has goals for the interaction which are not positive for their speech partner. For other examples, see (Barlow, 2021; Hewett et al., 2009; Lingard et al., 2004). These papers underline the intergroup nature of communication in the health context and how senior health professionals demonstrate their power through their communication style, both spoken and written.

Earlier in this chapter, I stated that making health providers aware of how their professional identities influence their interaction style and communication would assist in remedying problems of miscommunication. From my experience, when health providers learn about the principles behind social identity theory, they more often than not agree that their professional identity and relative status play a major part in how they communicate with others. That health providers recognise much of their work is actually about their professional identification and the hospital system suggests that they are able to reflect on their own roles and the roles of others, and on how they can be in conflict or in harmony. Given the complexity of the communication issues that health providers face, it makes sense to bring together diverse expertise to work with health practitioners. I have written elsewhere about three necessary steps for improving interprofessional health communication in order to make a difference (see Watson, 2020). These steps for researchers are to consult, to advocate and to use activism. The first two steps lead to action being taken, i.e., activism. Let me briefly discuss these first two steps. The third step is covered in Chapter 8.

All researchers must first learn to consult with all those engaged in healthcare: policymakers and administrators, as well as those health practitioners on the frontline. Too often, researchers bring their own particular theoretical perspective to a healthcare context and impose it on health professionals. They don't listen to what the health professionals have to say about what they think they need. Researchers must first invest time in discovering what health professionals believe are issues for them. Only then can both parties discover if together they can formulate a plan that addresses the needs of both, and assess how the researcher's theoretical framework may be best applied to each research context. But the concerns of the health professionals must always be the priority, not those of the researcher. Researchers sometimes impose their ideas on health providers because they know that health communication is a "hot topic". They want to obtain data without any real consideration of how health professionals and their patients may actually profit from any findings. Today's "publish or perish" mentality means that researchers are faced with enormous pressures, particularly the emphasis on obtaining competitive research grants and bringing money into their universities. These grants and the subsequent publication of their work are supposed to demonstrate their success as researchers. However, these pressures can prevent meaningful data from being collected (see Chapter 7 on research design and ethical issues).

The benefit of consulting with health professionals is that the researcher gets their side of the story and their perspective on a particular topic (e.g., handover). Research by Coupland et al. (1991) illustrates the likelihood that some health professionals may not envision other possible solutions or different ways of doing things. They are stuck in the traditions and cultures of the hospital system. Outside expertise can address how some activities can be changed, but it requires health providers to take the second step by advocating for the research necessary. To be an advocate within the hospital system demands that the research is significant to the health providers involved with the researchers, and this requires placing trust in the latter. Together, such relationships can produce outcomes that are meaningful. Health providers working in the hospital can become "insider champions", motivating others in the hospital to see the possibility of change. Insider champions can also actively challenge those who are resistant and can work to uncover the root cause of that resistance (Watson, 2020, see p. 185).

Review

In this chapter, I have overviewed how patient care is no longer a single doctor and patient situation. Many health providers can be involved in a patient's diagnosis and treatment. The GP organising a pathology test is a simple example of shared care. Hospital care as an inpatient can be one of the most complex. The message here is that numerous challenges arise for health providers, stemming from the organisational system of the hospital and its policy makers. Patient ownership and liaison between different specialists were targeted as a problem. But there is also the problem of individuals working within a system where their professional identity is highly salient for so much of the time. A senior doctor who wants to get their way to ensure their patient is treated before others will put pressure on colleagues to make it happen. They do not lack communication skills but rather use them to achieve their own goals. They want the best for their patient, but what happens to the other patients who have to wait? An intergroup perspective acknowledges this fact, helping pave the way to making existing issues more transparent.

Some Personal Review Points

- Can you recall any examples of when you felt it was difficult to communicate with someone honestly because of the difference in status or seniority? Who held the higher status, you or them?
- What would you like to see change when individuals, either in a multidisciplinary team or independently, share the care of a patient?
- Do you think the way you communicate encourages a sharing of ideas from others? If yes, why? If no, why not?

Healthcare Communication Across Cultures

Beliefs about illness and its causes differ across the world. This is still true in the twenty-first century. Taylan and Weber (2023) discuss their experiences of working with patients from diverse cultures. In their conclusion, they say:

> A trusting relationship between medical staff, patients, and their families does not necessarily require the ability to be fluent in every language, but the ability to listen to and observe people, if necessary, with the help of an interpreter. Projecting the feeling that the other culture is respected will make it easier for patients and their families to feel safe in the healthcare network. We often expect people from another culture to adapt to new conditions and to embrace the prevailing values, opinions, and traditions of their new homeland. However, this is often not the case as people hold on to their own values and it is important that we understand this instead of judging. The first step in this process can even be recognizing the problem as a problem. This awareness will optimize care and communication in one's own cultural bubble.
>
> Sometimes it is beyond language and just requires humanity (p. 648).

I believe they've got to the heart of this issue of how we can ensure effective intercultural health communication, and I'll develop some of their points in this chapter. Health professionals should be aware that a person's choice of treatment may often reflect their particular culture and their own beliefs about health. In our ever-changing and expanding global community, people from different countries with different languages and cultures are moving around the world more than ever before. These people represent different ethnicities, nationalities and geographic regions, as well as more specific aspects such as societal class, gender and profession (see Baker, 2024). Intercultural communication may be simply defined as communication between individuals coming from different cultures. To this basic two-word term, we add the word competence, implying that such communication will aim to be appropriate and ultimately successful.

I'm going to focus on the more traditional intercultural communication challenges that health providers face. I'll suggest that adopting an intercultural communication competence (ICC) perspective will prove insightful. As individuals move around the world, some will settle in cultures that will be distinctly different from those they have left. They may find it necessary to learn a second language and adapt to different ways of behaving in order to acclimatise themselves successfully to their new cultural environment.

The Challenges that Migrants Face in a New Country

How do migrants negotiate their lives elsewhere, having to deal with unfamiliar cultural norms and beliefs? They will inevitably vary in how well they acculturate to a new country, and there are numerous theories and approaches to explore intercultural communication and adaptation (e.g., Berry, 1997; Gudykunst, 2005; Kim, 2001). Much may depend on how and why the migrants arrived at their new destination, and the extent to which the host country has been chosen by them or forced upon them by local pressures. Migrants may well face discrimination from a host nation. They can be seen as a threat to national identity and economic well-being, taking jobs from host-nation members and becoming a drain on resources. In Hong Kong, domestic workers face a different type of discrimination. They can never be accepted legally as citizens, and they face healthcare challenges because of their dependence on their employers to support them. If they suffer ill-health, they may also face deportation (Turnbull & Wu, 2025; Wang & Watson, 2024).

The relationship between migrants and the host nation is a true ingroup and outgroup situation, one in which threat and conflict can be all too active components of the relationship. Discrimination by the host nation can take many forms. In 2023, The Guardian reported that half of all migrants who worked in Australia felt unsafe and had experienced bullying and verbal abuse (Convery, 2023). This report presented findings from a survey by The Migrant Workers Centre, which found that migrants were more likely to be discriminated against even though they possessed valid work visas, and that they often found themselves employed in insecure work or reporting to exploitative employers. Such bias reflects a conflictual and intergroup context for their living environment.

Almost all migrants will need to seek medical treatment at some time, but they will most likely be unfamiliar with how to access appropriate healthcare. Pattillo et al. (2023) reviewed the research on equity for migrants in their access to healthcare and found that active racism supports and strengthens healthcare inequalities. When migrants do need to make contact with a health service, they are faced with the problem of negotiating a whole new healthcare system. They may very well be disadvantaged. Research also shows that discrimination is detrimental to their health and well-being (Ziersch et al., 2020).

I'll discuss some of these challenges, in particular, two dominant traditions that communication researchers have applied to intercultural communication behaviour. The first is ICC, introduced initially in Chapter 4 (p. 49) in relation to interprofessional practice. The second is intergroup theory, which permeates this entire book. Each of these approaches focuses on different aspects of intercultural communication; each has its own specific advantages.

However, apart from the barriers to communication mentioned above, I noted in Chapter 4 that hospital patients often experience interactions with health providers as an intercultural experience. Thus, two layers of intercultural communication co-occur in the health context. Firstly, between patients and health providers as well as providers themselves, where at least one is from a different geographical region. Secondly within the hospital system itself, with its own culture and associated rules and norms. It's vitally important to recognise the complexity that these two inter-related layers of cultural challenge bring. Now it becomes possible to contrast the ICC training approach with the LSP perspective by investigating factors that the former doesn't take into consideration.

Dominant Research Traditions in the Study of Intercultural Communication

Background to the ICC Approach

I mentioned ICC and its emphasis on skills training when I discussed interprofessional communication in Chapter 4. Here I'll briefly describe the history of ICC and the context in which it was developed. An individual going overseas and experiencing a new culture will benefit by learning about their new environment in terms of its different cultural norms and social mores. In this way, the individual will be more likely to adapt and fit into their new environment. The ICC approach began with E. T. Hall, working with the American Foreign Service Institute to establish training programs for diplomats who would be posted overseas (Hall, 1973). These diplomats were required to know the social mores and rules of their host countries in order to work effectively and harmoniously there. The premise behind Hall's approach was that newcomers to a country should learn the language of their host country, as well as the local cultural norms and customs. Such training would ensure that diplomats become competent communicators.

This same philosophy has influenced health professionals who find themselves interacting with colleagues and patients from different cultures. The ICC training approach emphasises the interpersonal nature of communication. Skills are taught to help health professionals better manage conversations in an expanding global community, in which the number of incoming migrants continues to increase.

A paper by Schouten et al. (2023) provides an excellent overview of why such training is needed and how it can assist health professionals to communicate more effectively with culturally diverse populations. This training and its attendant philosophy suggest that when an individual interacts with someone from another culture, they may inadvertently say or do the wrong thing through ignorance. Learning new intercultural communication skills is a vital part of ensuring that effective communication will prevail, thus benefiting both the health professional who provides care and the patient who receives suitable and proper treatment. Nevertheless, researchers have noted some limitations with ICC.

Some Issues with an ICC Perspective

Kleinman and Benson (2006) observed that one problem is the way in which culture is defined by western countries. Specifically, they state that "Culture is often made synonymous with ethnicity, nationality, and language. ..... patients of a certain ethnicity – such as the 'Mexican patient' – are assumed to have a core set of beliefs about illness owing to fixed ethnic traits" (Kleinman & Benson, 2006, p. 1673). In other words, individuals from one nation stereotype those from different ethnicities or nationalities into groups and then specify each group's beliefs and traits. Kleinman and Benson (2006) provide examples of how bias and ethnocentric attitudes are harmful for good patient outcomes. Epner and Baile (2012) also demonstrate how early literature on cultural competence focused on categorising individuals by ethnicity, religion or national group (e.g., Hispanic or African American) and stereotyping them in this way. In line with Kleinman, they argue for the importance of recognising the needs of patients from a different culture by finding out what they actually think and believe.

Epner and Baile (2012) explicitly point out that associating an ethnic group with specific traits and beliefs is unhelpful. Such categorisation overlooks the fact that culture is dynamic and that a "one size fits all" attitude to a nation is completely inappropriate. They cite the work of anthropologists who have shown that culture is both dynamic and multidimensional, and go on to illustrate this point by providing case studies of four patients with advanced cancer, each from a different culture, who discover that they are no longer responding to treatment. Epner and Baile (2012) explain how each patient needed to be considered in a patient-centred way, their individual needs and beliefs listened to with empathy and respect. These differences are crucial for ensuring that each patient receives appropriate end-of-life care.

Contrasting ICC and Intergroup Perspectives

In contrast to ICC, an intergroup approach does not automatically assume that each speaker's ultimate goal is to achieve mutually effective communication in an encounter, even though collaborative communication may well be sought by each for part of the time. An intergroup communication approach addresses the challenges that exist when individuals experience prejudice or mistrust about other ethnic cultures. Social and historical relations between two cultures may give rise to negative perceptions by one or both speakers. The likelihood that the ICC principle of wishing to achieve a mutually effective interaction cannot, therefore, be assumed. For example, it's not hard to imagine conflictual communication between an Israeli and a Palestinian if they were to meet face to face. One or both might well experience a lack of goodwill, and might certainly not desire interaction.

Combining an ICC approach with an intergroup perspective allows researchers to explore how individuals' motivation and cognition can influence the effectiveness or otherwise of a conversation. Acknowledging that a person comes from an outgroup allows each speaker to be more aware of their differences and similarities. In this way, speakers can learn and understand what skills they require to assist them in conversing with individuals from other cultures. Relatedly, they can also gain insights into their own ethnocentric biases about a patient or a health professional. Combining ICC training with an LSP and CAT approach will provide insights into the patient's needs, concerns and understanding. As we'll soon see, ethnocentric attitudes to the management of healthcare treatment do exist and can seriously interfere with the rapport between health provider and patient. Relevant findings from CAT explicitly challenge the holding of stereotypical beliefs about someone from their appearance or origin. To make any assumptions about a patient based on where they come from is a sure recipe for miscommunication and poor patient outcomes.

I've discussed in earlier chapters that the application of CAT demonstrates how a person's sociohistorical background colours the way in which they initially orient themselves to an upcoming conversation with a health provider or patient (see Chapter 2). If this important dimension of how individuals differ in their beliefs and attitudes about healthcare is ignored or underrepresented, we risk losing important information. In turn, we then jeopardise our ability to explain how, in intercultural healthcare settings, communication is effective or ineffective.

I want to end this section about the dominant traditional approaches by citing the work of Professor Cindy Gallois. In her 2003 address as President of the International Communication Association (ICA) in South Korea, she emphasised the importance of recognising that intercultural communication is simultaneously interpersonal and intergroup. Not to actively acknowledge negative intergroup relations between groups is to ignore a fundamental aspect of the problem. She challenged all those who will work and research in intercultural communication by stating ".... ethnorelativism[3] is not enough. Trainers and trainees must think about and understand the impact of inequality, cultural domination, and the history of conflict on any encounter between individuals, no matter how well motivated they might be. To do this effectively, trainees need to clarify their own values and determine the ones that are not negotiable, so that they can work from a cultural anchor" (Gallois, 2006, p. 13). Gallois argued for recognition of all the many facets of intercultural communication training. Such training may reduce any negative attitudes that individuals hold about migrants.

Intercultural communication, as I've said, covers a wide range of topics. For this reason, I've found it necessary to be selective in the areas I discuss when I cover interactions between health provider and patient or exchanges between providers. Indeed, intercultural communication and healthcare could form a whole book in itself, but I have only this one chapter. Accordingly, I've carefully chosen research areas with which I'm most familiar in order to demonstrate the value of applying an intergroup LSP approach together with an ICC lens. For topics that I don't cover so fully, I provide a bibliography at the end of the chapter so that readers can find further information. I'll begin by exploring intercultural exchanges between health professionals and patients. This will clarify some of the difficulties that can arise when two speakers are not from the same geographic region and hold different cultural beliefs or values.

Intercultural Exchanges between Health Professionals and Patients

Different Beliefs about the Meaning of Illness, its Causes and Cures

Patients from different cultures may have very different understandings about what it means to be sick and how sickness should be treated. From a Western viewpoint, learning that other cultures have such diverse beliefs about sickness

---

[3] The perspective of understanding and respecting people's values and behaviours as culturally different rather than universal.

may seem strange. However, as noted nearly 50 years ago by the acclaimed anthropologist and psychiatrist, Arthur Kleinman, many other healing traditions exist outside of Western Medicine, and this still holds true today (Kleinman, 1978). The WHO has listed many types of traditional medicine, such as Chinese, Ayurvedic, Unani and homeopathy (World Health Organization, 2019b). In fact, 170 WHO Member States have confirmed that traditional medicine has been accessed among their populations. It isn't possible, nor is it necessary, to describe all of these healing traditions in detail. Rather, to illustrate my point, I will discuss just two. I'll describe how Western Medicine (WM) and Traditional Chinese Medicine (TCM) have different philosophies that result in different expectations and beliefs about illness and treatment. Although the one common theme across all traditions is an emphasis on being fit and healthy, we'll see that the concept of ill health can have very different meanings in other cultures.

WM can be described as an evidence-based biomedical model (Zhang et al., 2019). Historically, WM has developed by using organic substances such as herbs as antibiotics, and more recently, synthetically produced drugs, all of which are now rigorously tested for their efficacy. It is essentially a specific scientific approach. When a person is diagnosed with, say, breast cancer, the focus of treatment will be on that specific area of the body, while any signs of spread will be monitored. It is less likely that a holistic approach to contracting cancer will be considered beyond specific known risks. For example, WM explicitly demonstrates that there are links between cigarette smoking and lung cancer; accordingly, a health provider will advise a person with lung cancer to stop smoking. When an individual has a cancerous tumour, WM practitioners will seek to remove the tumour through surgery or reduce the tumour with chemotherapy or radiotherapy. In general, WM looks to find the source of a health problem and then focus on treating that location. WM practitioners are not especially versed in how various connections exist within the body, or that taking account of these can provide a very different picture of illness and disease. To explain this point further, let's now briefly examine some principles of TCM.

TCM has its roots in a very different philosophy. The brief paper by Zhang et al. (2019) discusses the fundamental differences between WM and TCM. In essence, Zhang and colleagues tell us that TCM takes an intuitive and traditional approach in that the particular combination of herbs prescribed for a patient is "personalized" for them. Treatment is not evidence-based like WM. That said, TCM is still a science. It has evolved over many centuries and is based on tested traditions. In TCM, an illness or disease signifies a lack of harmony within a person's body. Understanding that the body is an interconnected organism and must be treated holistically is a central belief. A more comprehensive account of

TCM is provided by Lozano (2014) in his chapter explaining its principles. He reminds us that TCM is at least 2000 years old, and that it assumes a person's health and their environment are connected. As Lozano states: "Disease is understood as a deviation from natural conditions, which correspond with changes in the natural environment. TCM thus describes diseases as being caused by wind, cold, dampness, heat, and so on, while the internal functions of the body are grouped together according to perceived systemic relationships" (p. 13).

For those unfamiliar with TCM, the premises put forward may seem esoteric and unscientific. However, we have only to look at how TCM provides us with intricate and detailed diagrams of human anatomy to see it as a serious and authentic healing tradition. I've personally experienced how pressure on one part of the body can correspond to sensations in another part of the body, which until then I'd seen as separate and unrelated. But in TCM, you cannot separate or isolate body parts – they are a whole. Certainly, more and more WM practitioners are looking to TCM as a complementary part of a patient's treatment. While living in Hong Kong for almost seven years, I became increasingly drawn to TCM and to an integrative approach between it and WM. An example of this approach in practice can be seen in the work of a colleague of mine, Dr Wendy Wong, a TCM doctor. Dr Wong is a specialist in colorectal cancer and a champion of integrative TCM-WM in which patients seek treatment from both (Wong et al., 2020). She and her team have worked extensively in this area, demonstrating that two disparate types of healing based on very different principles can be successfully combined.

Patient and Health Provider Explanatory Models

Arthur Kleinman found that people coming from different cultures may hold different explanatory models about the meaning of their own sickness (Kleinman, 1978). He showed that such individuals have differing understandings of what has caused their illness. This may have consequences for how they believe it should be diagnosed and treated. He also observed that if a doctor and patient have discordant beliefs about the underlying cause of a disease, it will very likely influence both how the initial medical interaction unfolds and the overall effectiveness of subsequent treatment. In some cases, treatment adherence can be compromised. Haidet et al. (2008) developed a tool to measure concordance and discordance between health providers' and patients' perspectives of illness. They called the tool CONNECT, a name they chose in order to lay stress on the importance of the health provider and patient being connected and in agreement. Haidet and colleagues expanded their research on explanatory models to include other reasons for different perspectives. Their work is a useful starting point for appreciating that discordant explanatory models may exist between health providers and patients because of their distinct cultural beliefs.

More recent research confirms that explanatory models should be seen as an important facet in patient treatment and care. Indeed, regardless of whether the basis for a discordant explanatory model between patient and health provider stems from cultural beliefs about what illness means or from some other reason, it can hinder patient outcomes if not detected. Thus, research again points to the need for recognition of a patient's individuality. It is imperative that the health provider be cognisant of the patient's explanatory model as well as their own, and incorporate the patient's beliefs into the treatment plan. It's perfectly possible for different explanatory models to exist side by side, and where necessary, the health provider may need to combine their own models with those of the patient to move the treatment forward (see Dinos et al., 2017).

Different Health Provider and Patient Health Expectations

Explanatory model discordance is not the only issue that health professionals and patients may face when they come from different cultures. As stated above, Kleinman and Benson (2006) emphasised how WM as a system of care can be extremely ethnocentric and biased, even when it purports to espouse cultural respect. This bias stems from the labelling of an ethnicity or culture as a set of homogeneous beliefs and behaviours, something we've seen to be unhelpful if health providers want to understand a patient's needs and perspectives on their illness. Taylan and Weber (2023) describe their experiences of working with patients from different cultures. They articulate the problems that occur when migrant patients interact with health providers who are not from the same culture, and when, because of this, different expectations may exist by each about how the actual communication process should play out. Taylan and Weber describe how some cultures expect or even demand patient-shared decision making and joint consultation, while others do not. Patients from cultures that don't normally encounter a collaborative approach may well be suspicious of the health providers' co-operative approach and sharing of information, seeing it as demonstrating inexperience or insecurity. In this scenario, patients expect doctors to direct them; making decisions for them regarding a course of treatment is their job.

The key issues and challenges facing both migrants seeking medical care and their health providers were reviewed in a concise and insightful paper by Schouten et al. (2020). The main concerns they listed centred around the provision of formal (professional) or informal (e.g., family) interpreters to assist in the consultation, an issue I will address in the next section of this chapter. Importantly, they also emphasised that language barriers were not the only challenge to intercultural health interactions; differences in cultural norms and values were another important part of this intricate puzzle. For example, health providers are increasingly encouraged to ensure patients participate and engage in shared decision-making. But, in some cultures, patients believe they should be passive participants; they do not want to assist in decisions about their treatment plan.

Research by Schinkel et al. (2019) clearly showed that Turkish minority groups living in the Netherlands neither expected nor wished to be part of a decision-making partnership with their doctors. They felt medical decisions were the remit solely of the physician. Schouten et al. argued that a holistic approach needs to be taken in which both language and cultural issues can be addressed. This would include the training of health providers in how to better understand migrant and ethnic minority patients, so as to become more informed about how they manage and negotiate patient care. They acknowledged it is a difficult task, while financial constraints alongside staff shortages make the problem of treating culturally diverse patients exceptionally demanding. Their paper demonstrates how these medical interactions cannot be viewed as solely interpersonal exchanges. Each speaker has a role to play, but the role that each believes they should adopt may not sit well with the other speaker. Other researchers have shown how clear and accurate communication between health providers and patients may be compromised (Isaacs et al., 2011; Segalowitz & Kehayia, 2011).

Isaacs and colleagues (2011) investigated the challenges that nurses faced when forced to use a second language while treating linguistic minorities. Their findings suggested that nurses found dealing with routine matters to be the least problematic, but that engaging with a patient on more emotionally charged issues, such as managing their negative feelings, was far more difficult. Nurses also found that providing information to a patient from a minority group by using a second language was challenging. The authors suggested that more attention should be given to the training of nurses who need a second language when working with patients. A paper by Segalowitz and Kehayia (2011) recommended that researchers working in language sciences investigate existing language barriers within healthcare. Their expertise would undoubtedly benefit both health professionals and patients who face such problems daily. Segalowitz and colleague's paper also highlighted the importance of an interdisciplinary approach where researchers from different disciplines work with frontline health professionals. This openness to sharing and collaborating in health communication research would, I believe, pave the way for innovative ways of managing these challenges, which health professionals alone may be unable to resolve without such outside assistance.

So far in this chapter, I've covered the bigger picture of intercultural dynamics and healthcare, discussing the ways in which health professionals learn about negotiating intercultural communication with their patients. I've shown that an ICC approach, while necessary and valuable, does have its limitations which, if ignored, can be detrimental to ensuring effective communication. I've mentioned the issues surrounding recognition of the uniqueness of individuals coming from other cultures, and I've shown how explanatory models may differ for patients and their health providers. In the next section, I'll examine in more depth the problems that emerge when both patients and health professionals from different cultures engage in health consultations.

Language Barriers between Health Professionals and Patients

A challenge that patients and health professionals from different cultures often face in a health consultation is that they don't speak the same first language. This means that neither the patient nor the health professional can easily communicate to identify the patient's health problem, the whole point of the exchange. When migrants cannot speak the language of the host nation, there may be delays in seeking and accessing medical treatment (Pandey et al., 2021). Pandey and colleagues found that as well as experiencing such delays migrants could not develop a therapeutic rapport with their health provider. Adherence to treatment was compromised through misunderstanding, leading to poor health outcomes. This situation represents a serious challenge for achieving clear communication between health provider and patient, a vital goal for both participants. The situation can be exacerbated when patients are highly anxious or afraid. Negative emotions are common enough in individuals familiar with the health context of their own culture; it isn't at all uncommon for them to feel uneasy about visiting a health professional in familiar surroundings (Baker & Watson, 2020). But an unfamiliar health setting with its own rules and norms is another hurdle for migrants to face. Al Shamsi et al. (2020) conducted a systematic review of the effects of language barriers. They found that such barriers are predictors of miscommunication and can result in a lower quality of patient care and reduced patient satisfaction.

Language barriers occur in varying degrees. In some instances, neither health provider nor patient has a shared language; in others, patients will speak the language of the host nation, though in varying levels of competency. As we saw earlier in this chapter, the extent to which migrants adapt to their host country depends on many factors. Some migrants never master the language of the host nation, others speak a little, and others again become fluent. For a discussion of why these differences occur, see Berry (1997). Where possible, it's beneficial for those migrants who cannot speak the host's first language to visit health centres where their own first language is spoken. This, of course, is by no means always possible. Zhao et al. (2021) investigated the extent to which members from minority groups experienced anxiety when they sought health treatment and were forced to use the host nation's language: their second language. They found that these minority group members experienced health anxiety because of this. In addition, compared to those seeking care for physical complaints, anxiety was more evident for those seeking support for their mental health.

Gasiorek et al. (2015) investigated how doctors working with patients who did not speak the same first language managed the language barrier during consultations. In this study, the doctors emphasised how important it was to use accommodative communication. They described patients as being fearful and distrustful when they could not understand doctors. At times, doctors would ask their fellow colleagues to assist them with the language, or they would attempt to use gestures to explain procedures. Doctors said they tried to show patients how contrite they were about the existing language barrier, and to impress on them that it did not affect their professional skills. This study also asked doctors to evaluate their levels of social distance (sense of connection and rapport) with patients. On this aspect, doctors reported that their sense of connection with the patient was higher when they perceived patient comprehension also to be high, but commensurately lower when patient comprehension appeared low. Findings also revealed that doctors recognised the importance of breaking down language barriers to encourage rapport with patients and reduce their anxiety. This study by Gasiorek et al. (2015) demonstrates clearly that ICC and an intergroup lens work hand in hand.

An intergroup LSP perspective acknowledges that the doctor is working as an expert from a specific professional group, tasked with caring for a patient. Their goal is to treat the patient effectively. Because the doctor is not competent to engage in accommodative verbal conversation with the patient, they try to provide reassurance (emotional expression) and clear explanations (interpretability) through non-verbal gestures. They combine their ICC training with what they believe to be accommodative communication strategies. The ICC training has educated the doctor about the different cultural beliefs and values the patient may hold. Ideally, what we would want is for the doctor not to categorise the patient as part of an ethnic group with set beliefs, but instead to recognise that they may have their own beliefs that should be investigated and respected. Such knowledge may well alert the doctor to the patient's sense of vulnerability. An intergroup LSP perspective provides the doctor with insights into the respective roles of each speaker. It should assist them in recognising the importance of employing accommodative communication strategies that are appropriate, in order to reduce the social distance between themselves and their patients.

The Use of Interpreters

If a patient, unable to speak the host language, needs to visit a health provider, it could well prove essential that someone else is present who speaks their language. One solution is to obtain the services of an interpreter, a person who could remove the communication barriers we've been describing. There is, in fact, a great deal of research into the use of interpreters going back more than 30 years (see Baker et al., 1996); it's clearly a multifaceted area still much researched. Dr Elaine Hsieh has demonstrated the complexities of this topic, covering many relevant issues of the communication dynamics present for patient, health provider and interpreter (Hsieh, 2016). However, obtaining an interpreter for a healthcare consultation is not an automatic process, and in many cases is not even considered simply because of the consequent delay to the patient's examination. A 2020 systematic review noted that the use of interpreters can increase the financial cost of patient services and extend a consultation's length of time (Al Shamsi et al., 2020).

The decision to use an interpreter often lies with the health professional. Jones et al. (2019) investigated this decision process in a study situated in a large tertiary hospital in Queensland, Australia. Their focus was on how health professionals decide if an interpreter is necessary. They conducted interviews with 69 health providers from a range of professions, all working in paediatric medicine. Most participants believed that it was the responsibility of the health professional to make the decision; it was not common for them to ask parents of the sick children if they wanted an interpreter. Overall, there was little uniformity in how these decisions were made. In line with Al Shamsi et al. (2020), Jones et al. also found that issues of time, availability and cost influenced the health professionals' decision making. Interestingly, health providers showed far more concern for the importance of family members to understand what a provider wanted to tell them than for what family members might want to know or relay to them. Use of an interpreter was restricted to information transmission by the health professional; any other nonmedical concerns were not thought sufficiently important. This research also suggested that some health professionals held stereotypical beliefs about some ethnicities. It is telling that the health professionals did not value the notion of a two-way communication between themselves and the family, and this again highlights issues that we've already discussed. The findings by Jones et al., certainly indicate a need for more training to take into account individual differences and individual needs.

From an LSP viewpoint, it is important to recognise that consultations including the presence of an interpreter will inevitably change the dynamics of the interaction: another person has become involved. Although interpreters are supposed to be merely the conduit for transmitting information, their presence will have a significant effect on the communication process and the development of any rapport. This should not be ignored. Two-way communication is vitally important – a three-way interaction will inevitably affect process and outcome. Elaine Hsieh (2006) used research findings on the use of interpreters in medical consultations to unpack some of the issues that arise when using different types of interpreter. Hsieh focused on how the employment of interpreters with differing skills could affect consultations. Her findings from the literature showed that ratings of positivity by health professionals for interpreter services were mixed.

Hsieh (2006) identified five types of interpreter employed during consultations: chance interpreters; untrained interpreters who worked with health providers in different roles; bilingual health providers; on-site medical interpreters formally trained in bilingual medical interactions; and lastly, trained telephone interpreters. Chance interpreters were usually family or close friends of the patient. Hsieh found that these were often rated positively by the patients and had their trust. However, family or friends might not always be a good choice. Children, for example, might be embarrassed about interpreting medical matters between health providers and their relatives, and might feel uncomfortable stepping outside of their normal social role. Relatives and friends might speak for the patient, but not translate fully what was said. In addition, they might not be sufficiently competent to provide an accurate translation.

Untrained interpreters as support staff in the medical environment might be more competent than family or friends, but their lack of medical training meant they were prone to interpretation errors. The use of bilingual healthcare providers was also not without problems. Hsieh cited research showing that being bilingual but formally untrained could mean that they failed to appreciate cultural nuances of the patient and might also overestimate their ability to understand what was being said. Hsieh then examined findings concerning on-site medical interpreters and telephone interpreters, both of whom had undergone some formal training. She noted that on-site interpreters were very expensive, and so medical facilities and hospitals might not be able to afford their services. Telephone interpreters had some advantages, but as they were not physically present, they obviously couldn't interpret any non-verbal communication. In sum, Hsieh found that on-site and telephone interpreters provided moderate to high quality interpretation, bilingual health providers varied more in ability, and both chance and untrained interpreters demonstrated low interpreting quality.

The use of an interpreter, then, does not necessarily provide the same level of information as a first-language patient receives. Butow et al. (2013) examined consultations between doctors and patients diagnosed with cancer. The patients were either Anglo-Australian speaking English or from overseas and not speaking

English. Their research showed that doctors did not vary their approach to explaining the prognosis of the cancer. How much prognostic information the overseas patients obtained was influenced by the presence of an interpreter. In these cases, twenty-three percent of the doctors' prognostic information was not relayed by the interpreter to the patient. Butow and colleagues' findings clearly indicate that much more needs to be done to remedy this potentially serious shortfall.

As I noted earlier, when a two-way consultation becomes necessarily three-way, the identity of the additional person can seriously affect the dynamic and ultimately the eventual outcome. The physical positioning of an interpreter is yet another important factor. The interpreter is the person whom both provider and patient speak to. Consequently, their precise location may lead to minimal verbal and nonverbal contact between the two main participants. Rapport and the patient's trust could well be reduced, leading to impairment of the communication process.

As you will appreciate, solutions to intercultural communication in healthcare are not readily available. This chapter cannot by itself provide answers to the problems raised. Rather, and in line with the appeal for a holistic approach to research and theory, it aims to expand the discussion by urging researchers to go beyond the ICC approach. Emphasising the argument of Cargile and Giles (1996), we can recognise the strengths in bringing together an ICC approach and an intergroup perspective. Sensitivity and respect for the patient's culture are essential components of the ICC perspective, but from an LSP approach, so too are the motivations and cognitions of both patient and health professional. Acknowledging these facts means recognising that some health providers hold ethnocentric views about other cultures and beliefs.

There is surprisingly little recent research on ethnocentrism or the cultural competence of health providers. Fisher (1992) emphasised that doctors must learn to communicate with their patients by making the effort to understand their perspective. Not to do so jeopardises their ever gaining a patient's trust, leading so often to miscommunication and non-adherence to treatment. Similarly, in another paper written over 15 years ago by Capell et al. (2008), the authors remarked that ethnocentricity and cultural competence were inversely related. Specifically, the higher a health professional's level of ethnocentricity, the lower their level of cultural competence. Thus, negative bias towards the beliefs of a particular culture may predispose the health professional to be dismissive of the patient's perspective. Broadening the scope of their cultural knowledge is therefore essential, given the rapid increase in persons from ethnic groups now seeking treatment.

One specific linguistic impediment to understanding for both first and second language speakers is worth special mention. Words such as "probably", "possibly", "likely" and "certainly" are frequently employed by health professionals in estimating a degree of perceived risk. However, these so-called epistemic adverbs are often understood differently depending upon the culture of the patient (Segalowitz et al., 2016). In order for health professionals to explain levels of treatment risk clearly and unambiguously, they must become aware that such adverbs can easily be misunderstood, resulting in patients – especially those from other cultures – misinterpreting the estimation of risk.

Intercultural Exchanges between Health Professionals

Thus far, I've concentrated on communication between health providers and patients whenever cultural differences and/or language barriers exist in consultations. I've also discussed the role of interpreters and how their presence is a critical aspect of health interaction in the way it can shape the communication dynamic, affect the information relayed, and influence possible adherence to treatment. I hope that the complexity of intercultural communication in healthcare is now very evident and that I've sufficiently demonstrated how taking an LSP and intergroup perspective opens up understanding and provides insights into the issues faced by both health providers and patients.

But what are the problems facing health professionals when they communicate with other professionals from different ethnic backgrounds? It could well be the case that there will be some lack of comprehension between first and second language speakers. It will certainly be the case that the cultural norms of the relative healthcare systems will differ. How much these cultural norms, language differences, and the past experiences of each health professional will affect working relationships is difficult to assess. Insofar as WM practitioners tend to be ethnocentric, their attitude to overseas health professionals working in the host nation may not be altogether positive. In Chapter 4, we saw issues that can arise when health professionals from different disciplines need to interact with each other. Now we have the further dimensions of nationality, ethnicity and cultural difference all requiring investigation.

In Chapter 4, I discussed how health professionals from different disciplines often use separate medical terms and how this can lead to misunderstanding, resulting ultimately in poor patient outcomes. In a rather different way, health professionals from the same discipline or sub-specialty, working with colleagues but from different cultural backgrounds, may hold divergent attitudes in some situations. An emergency department director once relayed to me some of the problems he faced when working with doctors from overseas. Some of these doctors, he said, were unwilling to break bad news to their patients. For these doctors, it was culturally inappropriate, and so they avoided the issue. He added that in a Western culture, it's now expected that patients and family would be told the complete truth about a diagnosis. Overseas doctors coming to a new culture need to be made aware of such important differences in communication practices. Such awareness would improve harmony between members of the host nation and overseas doctors.

Jalal et al. (2019) conducted a literature review that centred on how overseas doctors negotiated their transition to working for the National Health Service (NHS) in the United Kingdom, and on the difficulties they confronted. This comprehensive review went beyond communication challenges and dealt with the ever-changing administrative regulations that can make entry to the NHS more difficult for them. It showed that they are disadvantaged in that they cannot readily access important information that would assist and support them in their clinical practice. The findings of this review support the observation from the emergency department director that overseas doctors have great difficulty knowing how their host nation manages end-of-life decisions and the breaking of bad news. As we've seen, different cultures manage these issues in different ways. Jalal and colleagues' findings also revealed that the nonverbal communication of overseas doctors in terms of eye contact, facial expression and other body language may not align with the host nation's style of communication. Unfamiliar variations in nonverbal behaviour can be problematic for both other health professionals and patients. Indeed, these different styles of communication may be uncomfortable or even appear confrontational to the other person in a consultation.

It's telling that Jalal et al. (2019) found that bullying of both overseas and UK medical graduates was acknowledged to the same extent, but that overseas graduates were less likely to formally report such incidents. Their research illustrates a pervasive negativity in the hierarchical structure of the hospital that influences all junior staff regardless of culture. These findings should alert health professionals and health communication scholars to the problems that exist in the health system, which, I would suggest, are not peculiar to the United Kingdom (see bibliography at the end of this chapter).

Gasiorek and van de Poel (2012) investigated communication evaluations made by mobile medical professionals (MMPs) providing medical care in foreign countries where there are often different cultural norms and languages. They asked the MMPs to provide evaluations of their professional and social competency when interacting with native colleagues. They also asked the native colleagues to rate the competency of the MMPs. The MMPs reported that they believed their native colleagues perceived them to be competent communicators, but they also acknowledged that extra training with everyday language, as well as medical terms, would be helpful. The native colleagues valued the MMPs' contribution to health care highly, but reported a number of issues that they thought could compromise patient outcomes. These issues related to interactions with both patients and colleagues. Native colleagues rated the MMPs' communication as somewhat problematic in terms of their pronunciation, nonverbal communication, and use of small talk.

In contrast, the MMPs did not perceive any significant problems with their own communication. On the contrary, Gasiorek et al. made the important observation that the MMPs perceived themselves as effectively accommodating in a foreign context, based on their own beliefs of what signified appropriate communication behaviour. But, of course, their native colleagues were judging them from a different standard. The fact that the MMPs were unaware that their communication was sometimes inappropriate paves the way for continuing misunderstanding and miscommunication. Gasiorek et al. proposed that one way of reducing such failure would be by integrating ICC skills with an intergroup communication approach.

Al-Btoush and El-Bcheraoui (2024) conducted a review on the integration of migrant health care workers (MHCWs) across a number of quite disparate countries. Their review demonstrated that these new health providers experienced challenges with language, cultural adaptation and job satisfaction. The review also examined how likely it was that migrants would have intentions of remaining in the host nation and found that length of time was an important factor. Compared to migrants working in countries offering short contracts, such as Australia and Finland, those working in countries offering lengthier contracts, such as Sweden and the United States, were less likely to want to leave their new environment, as they had more career stability. Unsurprisingly, Al-Btoush and El-Bcheraoui (2024) emphasised the need for orientation programs and examination of the role that social isolation plays when MHCWs arrive in a new host nation. The review further found that migrants experienced difficulty in understanding new medical terms and in adapting to a new healthcare system.

And finally, actual job satisfaction was examined by Timilsina Bhandari et al. (2015). They surveyed 150 overseas-qualified nurses who had moved to Australia, some coming from English-speaking backgrounds and some from non English-speaking backgrounds. Nurses from non English-speaking countries were less satisfied and had shorter stays in Australia; they also reported experiencing discrimination and racism.

Review

This chapter has provided an illustration of some significant issues within the healthcare system that are related to cultural differences. I know that these issues are by no means unique to healthcare, but the ramifications for patients and for health professionals are clearly of considerable concern. An LSP approach by itself is insufficient to resolve these, but if LSP health communication scholars were to work with researchers from other disciplines and with the clinicians (i.e., health professionals) themselves, so much could surely be achieved.

Some Personal Review Points

- Have you considered how your beliefs about healthcare and treatment differ from other individuals? Do you think your own views are right?
- Can you think of any issues that have arisen when you have interacted with someone from another culture? This does not have to be a health-related incident.
    - What did you think was the problem? Was it resolved? If so, how was it resolved?
- Have any of your attitudes towards intercultural communication in the healthcare setting been challenged in this chapter? If yes, what are they?

Further Reading

Carlasare, L. E., & Hickson, G. B. (2021). Whose responsibility is it to address bullying in health care? *AMA J Ethics*, *23*(12), E931–936.

Kleinman, A. (1988). *The illness narratives: Suffering, healing, and the human condition*. Basic Books.

Kurylo, A. (2017). *Inter/cultural communication : Representation and construction of culture*. SAGE.

See also the following website: Bullying and harassment in the medical profession <https://www.aph.gov.au/Parliamentary_Business/Committees/Senate/Community_Affairs/MedicalComplaints45/Report/c03>

The Wicked Problem of the Healthcare System and its Influence on Communication

Two surgical patients were scheduled for an endarterectomy to treat peripheral vascular complications, requiring weight-based dosing of preoperative high-alert medications. Both patients were vastly different weights. During the preoperative interview, the nurse verified the medication orders and observed that both patients had high-risk medications in the manufacturer's packaging attached to their charts. The preoperative nurse opened the medication packaging and noticed that while the patient information was correct on the labels, the medication reflected the opposite patient's drug dosing. The preoperative nurse stopped what they were doing, called for an interprofessional safety huddle to verify the mistake, removed the incorrect medications from the area, and requested the correct medication dosage from the pharmacy.

(Stucky et al., 2024, p. 13).

This case study represents a near miss. A serious error was avoided through the preoperative nurse's prompt action. The authors of this paper state that much can be learned about reducing risk if we look at how near misses were spotted. This then is a good news story, but as we'll see, acknowledging the importance of near misses and providing praise for those who were responsible for avoiding error is not commonplace. In this chapter, I'll identify, through actual case studies, the complexities of healthcare that exist, and interpret events from an intergroup perspective. But let me start by explaining the rationale for the title of this chapter.

What Do We Mean by a Wicked Problem?

What is a wicked problem, and why have I chosen it as part of the title? Rittel and Webber (1973) discuss the properties of a wicked problem:

> ... we are calling them [problems] 'wicked' not because these properties are themselves ethically deplorable. We use the term 'wicked' in a meaning akin to that of 'malignant' (in contrast to 'benign') or 'vicious' (like a circle) or 'tricky' (like a leprechaun) or 'aggressive' (like a lion, in contrast to the docility of a lamb)? (p. 160).

I believe that the problems facing healthcare communication fit these descriptions of wicked very well. But do be clear that there is no malevolent objective implied for anyone involved in the wicked problem of healthcare communication. It's rather that the context is complex and requires the application of different approaches in order to improve the situation.

To quote Rittel and Webber again: "There is no definitive formulation of a wicked problem" (Rittel & Webber, 1973, p. 161). From this, we may infer that no single approach will necessarily fix anything. The authors suggest an analogy to street crime. There are, they say, many ways to explain this kind of crime: not enough police, too many criminals, deficient laws, too many guns available, cultural inequality, minority groups and so on. How do you tackle the problem of street crime? What is the best approach? How can we know? Street crime prevails despite the many efforts to reduce it. Similarly, in the health sector, money is thrown at more hospital facilities, improving aspects of healthcare and developing training interventions to assist health providers to work together, while programs for interprofessional education (IPE) are put in place in universities to ensure better shared communication. Yet, as this chapter will show, problems of miscommunication, safety, and quality healthcare continue. And so, when politicians or social policy workers come up with a solution to improve healthcare, it's almost always doomed to fail. If health providers and policy makers can be honest about the fact that healthcare and associated communication issues are wicked problems, then maybe a more meaningful dialogue can commence. Let's recognise that we need health economists, engineers in human factors, social scientists, social psychologists, linguists and others to collaborate with health providers working on the frontline. Hospital policy makers and senior management must also be involved. This need for closer collaboration, a major running theme throughout this book, I'll address in more detail in Chapter 8.

I'm going to describe some specific events that led to patient harm, all of which occurred in the hospital system. These events had various causes, but communication and the intergroup environment within healthcare are shown to be significant contributing factors. In previous chapters, I've discussed how health professionals communicate with each other and their patients in order to ensure quality patient treatment and care. I hope by now it's becoming increasingly clear that healthcare contexts, especially the hospital environment, are indeed complex. This complexity, as I pointed out in Chapter 4, is due in part to the multifaceted role of health providers. I said there that different professions must work together to manage the care of individuals who often suffer from comorbidities. We saw that health providers frequently work in circumstances that are less than ideal. Clinicians must compete for limited resources, and not everyone can get what they need to give the best care for their patients. Limited resources mean that conflicts arise between departments, such as between the emergency department and hospital wards. Stories of corridors filled with patients waiting to be seen in the emergency department or waiting for a bed on a ward are now commonplace (e.g., Sartini et al., 2022; Savioli et al., 2022). I also discussed in Chapter 4 how health professionals work long hours, have a great deal of responsibility, and frequently have to shoulder this responsibility when they are still quite junior. All this co-occurs in a hospital environment which is typically bureaucratic, with a hierarchical structure in which the power and status of doctors is paramount. Such conditions invite miscommunication, which in turn can often lead to patient harm. When a patient experiences such harm, it is known as a sentinel event.

Sentinel Events

There have been increasing concerns about the number of avoidable incidents of patient harm occurring in hospitals, and it has become an urgent priority for health services (Garzon Gonzalez et al., 2023; O'Connor et al., 2023; Umberfield et al., 2019). What precisely do we mean by the term "incident"? The WHO states: "An incident can be a reportable circumstance, near miss, no harm incident or harmful incident (adverse event) .... A *harmful incident (adverse event)* is an incident that results in harm to a patient (e.g., the wrong unit of blood was infused and the patient died from a haemolytic reaction)" (World Health & Safety, 2010, p. 16). We may compare this to the following: "Sentinel events are a subset of adverse patient safety events that are wholly preventable and result in serious harm to, or the death of, a patient" (Australian Commission on Safety and Quality in Health Care ACSQHC, 2020, p. 5). It is clear that the terms adverse and sentinel are closely connected, and in fact their meaning and reference can overlap across different countries and health organisations. For this reason, and for consistency, I shall use the term sentinel event to refer to all events that have led to some level of patient harm.

The incidence of sentinel events is high across the world and, more importantly, it is not significantly decreasing (*The joint commission sentinel events data*

2023 annual review, 2024; Panagioti et al., 2019). In 1996, The Joint Commission established a Sentinel Event Policy. For 2022, it reported a 19% increase over 2021 in such events, identifying a prime factor, as in earlier years, to be communication breakdowns. But there is no one reason for their incidence. The World Health Organization (2017) has noted that:

> Medication errors can be caused by health worker fatigue, overcrowding, staff shortages, poor training and the wrong information being given to patients, among other reasons. Any one of these, or a combination, can affect the prescribing, dispensing, consumption, and monitoring of medications, which can result in severe harm, disability and even death.

Because we are human, errors will occur, and they will often be due to the reasons given by the WHO. The 1999 Institute of Medicine (IOM) report heightened awareness of this whole issue when it stated that medical error ranked eighth in causes of death in the United States (Institute of Medicine Committee on Quality of Health Care in, 2000; Wakefield, 2000). This report garnered much attention at the time, and this attention has not diminished in the years since. Discussions of this topic have extended to related issues, e.g., clinicians not wanting to admit to failures for fear of losing their reputation with other health professionals and with future patients, or the financial and emotional costs of litigation (Lucian L, 2009; Vogus et al., 2010).

However, the relationship between avoidable patient harm and communication failure has been consistently acknowledged as a critical factor (Guttman et al., 2021; Kwok et al., 2020; Sutcliffe et al., 2004; Watson & Wu, 2022). Biquet et al. (2021) provided a comprehensive review of the complexities associated with ensuring a culture of patient safety. They emphasised that a blame culture is clearly not conducive to active error reporting. Management should be encouraging a culture in which reasons for errors are recognised, so that the errors themselves become a learning tool for ensuring non-recurrence. Brattebo and Flaatten (2023) examined sentinel events and concluded, in line with the WHO, that there are many factors to consider. The hospital represents a complex system that in some ways has a life of its own. Any changes to the system can, for good or ill, affect other parts of the system, and these effects are not always foreseen or immediately recognised. The topic of sentinel events could easily form a book by itself, but my particular aim here is to link these events to the intergroup dynamic of the hospital workplace and its attendant communication behaviour. Awareness of this intergroup dynamic may assist health providers and management in becoming more aware of the factors governing errors, so that they may then find new ways of substantially reducing their frequency.

Previously Reported Sentinel Events

There are numerous examples of sentinel events, though not all have led to permanent harm or death. You will see that those I'm going to describe are quite diverse, and while communication and the intergroup dynamic are present in all of them, other factors are also relevant. Each example represents a wicked problem. Regrettably, there is no one solution for such distinct problems, but I would argue that if we understand that we are dealing with complexity and multifaceted issues, this will open up a dialogue for more collaboration across scientific disciplines, as well as with health professionals and hospital management. I shall first describe one specific sentinel event that was widely reported in Queensland, Australia, and which illustrates how patient care can be compromised by a team of health professionals. My second example concerns a number of closely related sentinel events that took place at one hospital. Although both examples occurred some time ago, numerous other more recent events demonstrate that such problems still exist (*The joint commission sentinel events data 2023 annual review, Sentinel events statistics 2024. <http://www.Jointcommission.Org/sentinel_event.Aspx>*). As I write this book, research is continuing into the case of the neonatal nurse, Lucy Letby, convicted of murdering babies in the neonatal intensive care unit at the Countess of Chester Hospital in the United Kingdom. A BBC article (<https://www.bbc.com/news/articles/cx2y5zqw0jdo>) reported concerns over communication between the hospital director and the coroner's court. The heading on the BBC webpage for 5 December 2024 stated: "Coroner not told of Letby concerns, inquiry hears". The last section of this report read as follows:

> Mr Moore, who replaced Mr Rheinberg as senior coroner in March 2017 and retired himself in June 2022, added: "The provision of timely, accurate and truthful information is fundamental to the coronial process.
>
> "If the Countess of Chester had become aware of any information which had not already been disclosed to the coroner's office that would impact upon a death, the Countess of Chester would have been required to disclose that information immediately.
>
> "The Countess of Chester would have been expected to notify the police immediately if it had any reason to suspect that a person or persons may have been criminally responsible for causing a death.
>
> "The coronial process is a judicial process. It demands complete candour from healthcare professionals, clinicians, nurses and from hospital staff and also from trust management.
>
> "A failure to disclose to the coroner any information which may have a material bearing on a coronial case, whether it's been through the coronial process already or is pending, is to mislead the coroner and to mislead the court."

> Letby, 34, from Hereford, is serving 15 whole-life orders after she was convicted at Manchester Crown Court of murdering seven infants and attempting to murder seven others, with two attempts on one of her victims, between June 2015 and June 2016.
>
> The inquiry, sitting at Liverpool Town Hall, is expected to sit until early 2025, with findings published by late autumn of that year.

It would be improper to speculate about this case before the report is completed, but it isn't unreasonable to suggest that this will, in all likelihood, be seen as a highly involved matter with intergroup dynamics playing a conspicuous role.

I'll begin by describing some past events with which I am familiar, and which will allow me to apply an intergroup perspective. I'll then go on to examine a wider range of events that took place in public hospitals in Hong Kong. These are more recent and are representative of the types of everyday events that occur in hospitals elsewhere. The fact that they are so common is a worrying statistic that must not be ignored. The question we are investigating here, but return to in Chapter 8, is simply this: How can we fix the wicked problem?

Ryan Saunders - Australia

The first sentinel event I want to describe to you occurred in 2007. Although much time has passed since then, the general circumstances that led up to this event are as much in evidence today. The State Coroner's findings are the basis for the information reported (Barnes, 2011). On 20 September 2007, the mother of three-year-old Ryan Saunders took him to their GP, who incorrectly diagnosed mumps. In the early hours of 24 September, Ryan's mother called an ambulance because her son was in pain, despite taking common medication. Ryan was seen at the local hospital's emergency department, where tests were ordered. Doctors decided that Ryan needed an abdominal ultrasound, but this could not be conducted there. (The subsequent coroner's report stated that independent experts judged Ryan's treatment by the local hospital as appropriate.)

Ryan was airlifted to Rockhampton Base Hospital in Queensland, arriving there at 4:48 pm on 24 September, so that he could have the abdominal ultrasound. The consultant (the senior doctor in charge) diagnosed a viral infection, meaning that antibiotics used for treating bacterial infections were not administered. Over the course of the next 31 hours, the cause of Ryan's pain remained unresolved. One doctor recommended a test for a bacterial infection, but this request was declined by the consultant, who remained convinced that Ryan's problem was viral in nature. This doctor accepted the consultant's ruling, later stating that to approach a higher authority within the hierarchy in order to override the consultant was not something they felt they could do, and that, in any case, no clear pathway for such a course of action existed. In addition, Ryan's pain was not being well-managed, and the consultant refused a request by the same doctor to give morphine, even though other pain relief medications were proving ineffective. The consultant's justification for this decision was that morphine could mask the actual location of the pain. However, upon a further request by other medical staff later that day, he did finally prescribe morphine.

In the early evening, after another doctor had seen Ryan and noted his deterioration, it was decided that he should be flown to Brisbane. In preparation for the journey, Ryan needed to be intubated and ventilated. At 11:28 pm on 25 September, Ryan was successfully intubated, but shortly after suffered a cardiac arrest. At 11:40 pm, a medical emergency team arrived to attempt resuscitation, but their efforts were unsuccessful, and CPR was stopped at around 12:15 am on 26 September. The autopsy report stated Ryan's cause of death as "Group A Streptococcal Toxic Shock Syndrome" (Barnes, 2011, p. 19). The coroner, Michael Barnes, determined that "Ryan died from toxic shock after those treating him failed to detect and respond to the infection in a sufficiently timely manner" (p. 19). He noted that although the consultant was experienced, he often had to work with "inadequate resources and limited support" (Barnes, 2011, p. 20). Nevertheless, he concluded that the consultant should have been more aware of Ryan's condition and ordered more tests.

As a direct result of this most distressing case, the Health Quality and Complaints Commission made a number of recommendations, including "a review of communication within the healthcare team in the Paediatrics Unit at Rockhampton Hospital". This review was subsequently carried out, commenting on "areas such as patient handover; communication between staff and appropriate escalation of clinical management issues" (Barnes, 2011, p. 32). When reading the coroner's comprehensive report, it becomes clear that the medical team did not communicate successfully with the consultant and felt unable to challenge his opinion. While poor resources and long working hours must also be considered, the power dynamics and the intergroup hospital culture prevented action that might well have saved Ryan's life. It would appear that other doctors could not voice disagreement with the consultant strongly enough. We've already seen that such reticence is part of an intergroup hospital culture.

Dr Jayant Patel

The sentinel events related to Dr Jayant Patel, who became known in Queensland as "Dr Death" (Dunbar et al., 2011), also go back some time. For Australia, his story began in 2003, although his misdemeanours predate this year; a search on social media will quickly yield past details. And for those interested, a book covering the story of Dr Patel's outright neglect of his patients is available (Dunbar et al., 2011). Dr Patel was Director of Surgery at the Bundaberg Hospital in Queensland between April 2003 and April 2005. The sentinel events that occurred while he was in tenure led to a full overview of the Queensland Health System. I've chosen to draw on the report by Queensland Public Hospitals Commission of Inquiry released in November 2005, headed by the Honourable Geoffrey Davies AO QC (Queensland Public Hospitals Commission of Inquiry, 2005). These events are therefore a matter of public record. The report also covers other Queensland hospitals, but my focus will be solely on the Bundaberg Base Hospital and Dr Jayant Patel. I don't intend to outline all the negligent acts of this doctor – there really isn't space. My purpose is to highlight once again the hierarchical and intergroup nature of much of the healthcare system and its communication failure.

The Bundaberg Base Hospital faced budget shortages; Queensland Health was not responsive to budgetary expansion. The report provided a background of too much bureaucracy from the administration, leading to powerlessness on the part of medical staff. The reader will be aware that this represented a serious conflictual intergroup situation. Requests for more medical staff were dismissed by Queensland Health; senior clinicians resigned because of their frustration at not being able to deliver appropriate services. There were clearly a number of background issues around the management of the hospital and its ability to provide quality care. The end result was that Dr Patel arrived at the Bundaberg Base Hospital to take up a position he was not qualified to hold.

He was recruited as Director of Surgery in 2003. Mistakes were made in the checking of his resume, and Dr Patel himself concealed that he had been unemployed immediately prior to accepting this position. The Medical Board of Queensland did not follow the full procedure for verifying his credentials. If they had, it would have come to light that his Certificate of Licensure from Oregon, USA, contained a restriction on the types of surgery he could perform, and also that he had surrendered his licence to practise in New York. Effectively, he slipped through the net. The Director of Medical Services, Dr Keating, did not conduct any skills assessment, a prerequisite for such an appointment to the hospital. Dr Keating was found negligent in this regard. Three doctors at the Bundaberg hospital were aware of Dr Patel's deficiencies as a surgeon. One of the doctors, Dr de Lacy, stated in the official report that:

(a) His assessment of a presenting patient was inadequate;
(b) His surgery techniques were defective;
(c) His post operative management was poor; and
(d) His follow-up was inadequate.

> He concluded by saying that Dr Patel's results "were not ten times worse than one would expect; they were one hundred times worse" (p. 3).

The second doctor stated that he most certainly would not allow Dr Patel to operate on him. The third, Dr Woodruff, said that Dr Patel's poor level of care led to 13 patient deaths, and that a further four could be associated with his care. Thirty-one patients had experienced patient harm in varying degrees at his hands.

These are manifestly most damning statements. One wonders how Dr Patel was able to have his contract renewed, and how he could possibly have been awarded the accolade of employee of the month in November 2004. This award was in recognition of his ability to conduct a high number of surgical procedures on patients. One explanation is that the hospital, like most hospitals to this day, was run as a business with a fixed hospital budget. Keeping to budget was in practice more important than patient care and safety. In fact, the District Manager, Mr Leck, had been in danger of being sacked if he did not meet budget targets. The report also stated that the complaints system was woefully inadequate. Both Dr Keating and Mr Leck failed to comprehend that there were too many complaints about Dr Patel, some extremely serious, for them to ignore (Queensland Public Hospitals Commission of Inquiry, 2005).

On page one of the report, the Commissioner of the Inquiry, Geoffrey Davies, stated:

> Those complaints and concerns might never have been made public or been properly addressed if it had not been for the efforts of three people. The first and most important of these was Ms Toni Hoffman. It was her courage and persistence which, in the face of inaction and even resistance, brought the scandalous conduct of Dr Patel to light.

The fact that such shocking breaches of patient safety by one doctor might have gone unreported says much about the culture of the Bundaberg hospital, and from other more recent sentinel events that have occurred elsewhere, it's clear that such a culture is by no means uncommon (World Health Organization, 2023).

Ms Toni Hoffman, a senior nurse at the hospital, raised concerns with management about Dr Patel but was being constantly ignored. It took a member of the Queensland Parliament – Mr Rob Messenger, MP – to take up Ms Hoffman's case in Parliament before any action commenced. He was the second important person to bring Dr Patel to public attention. The third was a journalist with the Brisbane Courier Mail daily newspaper – Mr Hedley Thomas. The Commissioner called Dr Patel's conduct "appalling": a serious indictment of the health care system at the Bundaberg Base Hospital. Interested readers can seek further details of the many separate cases either from the book mentioned above (Dunbar et al.,

2011) or the book by the journalist (Thomas, 2007). So, what actually happened during those two years from April 2003?

I'll describe just one case, representative of the sentinel events caused by Dr Patel, in some detail. It concerned a Mr James Phillips. He was suffering from a lesion in his oesophagus, which accordingly required its partial removal. Mr Phillips was on renal dialysis, which further complicated the surgery. This type of operation is considered difficult even without the added complication of the patient's renal condition. It would therefore have been more appropriate to transport Mr Phillips to a larger tertiary Brisbane hospital. Nevertheless, Dr Patel performed the operation, and the patient was transferred to intensive care for treatment. It was there that Nurse Toni Hoffman encountered the patient. At the inquiry, she stated that Mr Phillips was very unstable when he presented at intensive care, with a blood pressure so low that it could not be recorded. Because of the need for dialysis, the doctors treating him could not all agree on the treatment plan. Mr Phillips eventually died in intensive care. Ms Hoffman was very concerned about the case and reported it to her line manager. Both the line manager and Ms Hoffman made an appointment to see Dr Keating. At this meeting, Ms Hoffman asserted that Dr Patel displayed a rude manner to staff and did not work collaboratively with them. She had also observed that his knowledge was outdated. She later stated to the Inquiry that during the meeting she had:

> [I].....attempted to paint an overall picture of the problems we were encountering in the Intensive Care Unit with Dr Patel including our observations as to the way Dr Patel interacted and spoke which indicated that something was not right. I also recall advising that Dr Patel appeared to be very old fashioned in his treatments...I recall Dr Keating saying that we had to allow that Dr Patel was from another country. I specifically recall advising Dr Keating that it was more like we were coming from two different planets (Queensland Public Hospitals Commission of Inquiry, 2005, p. 100).

Ms Hoffman was concerned that Dr Patel had been telling Mr Phillips' family that he was stable, which was inaccurate. She also made the point that for this type of operation, the hospital had inadequate facilities for appropriate patient care.

Other sentinel events included wrong-site surgery and problems with wound care as Dr Patel did not wash his hands between patients. Of special note is the fact that nurses were continually "trying" to get Dr Patel to wash his hands between patients, but he commented to them that "Doctors don't have germs", (Queensland Public Hospitals Commission of Inquiry, 2005, p. 111). In sum, there were over 20 complaints about Dr Patel during the 24 months of his employment at the Bundaberg Base Hospital. No competence checks were made on his skills during that period. Especially worrying, after so many complaints were voiced, was that only one doctor at the hospital directed that Dr Patel should not carry out surgical procedures on his own patients.

There is enough information here to suggest that Dr Patel should not have been allowed ever to practise in Queensland; he should have been forced to discontinue very early on during his time in Bundaberg. That this did not happen highlights the many problems that the hospital faced with budget shortages, poor resources and a management that did not take action because the whole situation would have reflected badly on them. Mr Leck would have lost his job. This whole situation demonstrated a lack of ensuring quality patient care and emphasised factions and conflict within the hospital, the hospital system, and even the Queensland State Government. It represented a wicked problem that did not have one simple solution. Doctors were complicit in working around Dr Patel. The report suggested that staff were demoralised and felt helpless in the face of the havoc that Dr Patel was wreaking,

Sentinel Events in Hong Kong Public Hospitals

In this section, I want to illustrate that sentinel events are by no means a problem unique to the Western World. Asia also experiences many such similar instances. While in Hong Kong, I investigated the incidence of sentinel events that the Hospital Authority (HA) there had disclosed in their annual reports (Watson & Wu, 2022). My colleague, Ivy Wu, and I examined these for the 43 Hong Kong Public hospitals. The HA classifies sentinel events into nine categories, representing different types of incidents. These include surgical procedures to the wrong patient or body part, instruments or other material retained in the patient after surgery, and errors leading to permanent loss of function or unexpected death. Our Hong Kong study confirmed that the reported events were comparable to those occurring in other Western hospitals.

As well as categorising events by type, the HA also analyses them by degree of severity. Other similar severity indexes are used around the world in the health sector. To grade the outcome of an event, a combination of descriptors such as "insignificant", "minimal", "mild", "minor", "moderate", "major", "severe" or "extreme" is employed. These show that not every event has disastrous consequences. Yet we should not be at all complacent about the lesser outcomes of effects graded as, for example, "insignificant" or "minor". All events are indicators of a problem. The fact that some don't result in permanent loss of function or death is obviously most fortunate, but this shouldn't obscure the need to investigate all of them. The Hong Kong HA uses a five-point index ranging from "insignificant" (meaning that no actual injury was sustained) to "extreme" (signifying major permanent disability or death).

Our study began by examining the 379 sentinel events reported for the period from October 2007 to September 2117. From this database, we eventually identified 186 events in which it was evident that miscommunication had been a contributing factor. This finding confirms much of the literature I've cited that identifies communication failure as an important factor in the occurrence of sentinel events. See: <https://www.safetyandquality.gov.au/sites/default/files/migrated/APPENDIX-B-International-sentinel-and-never-events.pdf>.

To capture as many forms of communication as possible, we categorised it into seven modes. We used three single modes, "spoken only", "written only" and "system-related only" (i.e., reflecting communication via a computer system), and four combinations of these (Watson & Wu, 2022). Of the seven modes we'd identified, "spoken +written" was the most prominent communication mode, accounting for 92 (49%) sentinel events, with "written only" representing a further 65 (35%). Because of their prevalence, we concentrated our study on these two.

The most commonly occurring event was surgical items retained in the patient after a procedure: a total of 116 events, of which 33 (28%) were graded as causing moderate or major patient harm. This was followed by procedures on the wrong patient or wrong body part, of which there were 44 incidents, 33 involving surgery or intervention procedures on the wrong site and 11 involving procedures on the wrong patient. To discover more about these two types of event and the factors reported to be associated with them, we examined the section in the reports concerning the investigation conducted by the hospitals involved. Unlike the cases of Ryan Saunders and Dr Patel that led to public investigations, the usual course of action after a sentinel event has occurred is for the hospital itself to conduct a root cause analysis (RCA). We need to examine this RCA method of inquiry.

RCA Identified Factors

The "written only" communication mode was largely concerned with documentation and guidelines or protocols in sentinel events. For wrong patient or body part and retained surgical items in patients, the RCA found that written communication broke down because information relayed was ineffective, being either inaccurate or inefficient. Specific causes included inaccurate reporting of the number of gauzes used in a procedure, unclear instructions or prescription orders, and information that was not up to date. RCA reports stated that health professionals performed treatment or procedures without giving attention to the patient's medical notes. In one example, a nurse assumed one piece of gauze had been placed in a patient's vagina when reference to the notes would have shown two. Only one was removed. Another problem concerned inaccurate communication about the specific operation site of patients, potentially resulting in wrong-site surgery. Written information played a role in some drug prescriptions where orders or request forms were unclear. In one incident, the RCA report noted that the instruction for a patient to receive a reduced dosage of a medication, because they were at high risk of cardiac failure, was obscured by the patient's label on the actual request form. The patient, therefore, received the regular adult dose and six days later died. Key written information for guidelines and protocols was not always relayed from hospitals to health providers. Such miscommunication can have many causes: multitasking, fatigue or simply poor handwriting. It does not always uniquely target an intergroup context.

"Spoken + written" information incidents provided more insights into how sentinel events are associated with the hospital hierarchy and power status differentials. As with "written only", this mode also included retained instruments or material in patients. Seventeen were classified as minor and five as having moderate or major patient harm outcomes. Nine gauze retention incidents under this mode occurred in the intraoperative period. The RCA investigation into events that led to patient harm again noted that causal factors included unclear or inaccurate documentation, but it also reported that spoken communication between members of the surgical team was not optimal. Specifically, for wrong patient or body part incidents, the team used closed questions or did not verify the patient's identification before commencing the procedure. Especially worrying was that often when a team member did realise there was a problem, such as an instrument unaccounted for, they did not actually voice their concern. However, in two incidents, the RCA report stated that the nurses alerted doctors about a missing gauze but were ignored, and that "these incidents occurred because of the surgeons' low awareness of retained gauze and their lack of response to the nurses' concerns" (Watson & Wu, 2022, p. 6). These events demonstrate how it remains the case that nurses are ignored and the hierarchy prevails.

RCA Recommendations

The Watson and Wu (2022) paper also examined the scope of the RCA recommendations. When I've spoken to health providers over the years, they've often remarked on how ineffectual these recommendations are. I wanted to follow this up. At one hospital where I conducted research, doctors openly voiced their opinion that RCA recommendations were, for most of the time, of no use. As I was working on communication-related sentinel events in Hong Kong, this presented an ideal opportunity to explore the recommendation process for the events that I had investigated.

The recommendations for the "written only" sentinel events included the redesigning of forms and the regular revision of records and checklists, the placing of a stronger emphasis on clear written information from hospitals, and a more rigorous enforcing of staff compliance with guidelines and protocols. However, these recommendations were not based on any investigation into why compliance might be lacking or whether non-compliance was ever intentional.

The recommendations for "written + spoken" were very specific to the events. Firstly, health professionals should be more willing to speak up when they recognise issues that need to be addressed. Secondly, they should liaise more actively with professionals from other disciplines. Thirdly, junior health providers should ensure that they consult with senior professionals as needed. And fourthly, health professionals should be more team-focused so that missing instruments are regarded as a joint responsibility. The RCA reported that health professionals did not seem to work in a coordinated manner when they were faced with larger team situations, and that clear role delineation was needed for each team member. While all the recommendations for "written only" and "written + spoken" may be pertinent, we must ask the crucial question: How will these changes be brought about? I here refer you to Chapter 4 on interprofessional communication and the events described there.

When we investigated the value of these recommendations in our 2022 paper, we were keen to explore whether the RCA teams concentrated only on the immediate circumstances of the events, or whether they also examined peripheral or antecedent factors that might have had relevance or that could be associated with them. Given the complexity and hierarchical structure of the hospital system, looking beyond the immediate circumstances might very well offer more insights into how incidents actually unfolded. Regrettably, we found that the RCA teams had directed their attention only to actions and behaviours that had occurred at the moment of the incidents, this focus being reflected in the nature of their recommendations. While this attention is clearly critical, it does mean that other potentially relevant factors that might have occurred beforehand were not considered. Recommendations concentrated on teaching staff communication skills, such as speaking up or learning to work better as a team. These are sensible as far as they go, but are too closely tied to the immediate circumstances and so don't fully address precisely how or why the events occurred.

When events consistently repeat themselves, it becomes necessary to look outside of the immediate circumstances for other patterns of behaviour that might be linked to them and which could provide further, vital information regarding causality. This lack of insight by RCA teams has not gone unnoticed by researchers investigating the efficacy of RCA recommendations. In our study, we noted that RCA teams mentioned staff shortages only once and alluded to staff inexperience only six times. Given the many challenges that health providers face in the hospital system, it's apparent that the focus on improving training is only one small part of the answer. Insufficient staff or regularly having inexperienced staff in charge, especially during night duty, needs more attention. So, what are the problems with the current RCA system?

Criticisms of RCAs

The RCA procedure has often been criticised because unlike, for example, aviation disasters, investigations into sentinel events are not conducted by an independent body. Thus, there is often a perceived conflict of interest (Kellogg et al., 2017; Percarpio et al., 2008). Clinicians are trained to focus on patient problems and to solve them. Nurses tend to see a bigger picture around patient care. These observations are generalisations, but they nevertheless sum up recognised differences between the two professions (see Vreugdenhil et al., 2023). I discussed in Chapter 4 how these two professions train separately and have their own cultures. What I believe impedes the success of RCA investigations is that they are internal and do not have independence or expert knowledge provided from other disciplines. Peerally et al. (2017) allude to these very problems, as well as raising their own important concerns regarding the RCA process. The notion of a health system that is hierarchical and essentially intergroup is not explicit in their paper. However, that said, we can place an intergroup lens on their observations. Doing so provides another insight into why RCAs are not reducing sentinel events.

Sentinel events are wicked problems. Peerally et al. (2017) make a number of observations, and I highlight a few here. They note that one problem lies in the name "root cause analysis" as the term for investigating problems. It suggests that "a single root cause (or a small number of causes) can be found", and as such suggests a reductionist perspective (Peerally et al., 2017, p. 417). Often, and as my examples and those of other researchers have shown, that is a false premise. Their second observation concerns having in-house health providers conduct the investigation. I've already shown how time-poor clinicians are. To be drawn away to investigate a sentinel event is not a welcome task, and health providers, while anxious to find out what happened, may also want to protect their colleagues. The authors also note that there may not be support from senior management for any suggested implementations. One obvious reason for resistance could well be the prohibitive cost. In essence, the paper suggests that in-house health providers are not equipped to investigate sentinel events effectively.

My own research has found that the challenge lies in ensuring health professionals are made aware of the contexts in which they interact, and that they see antecedent behaviour as equally important to monitor, and to question it where appropriate. Researchers from other disciplines, including communication, can and must actively seek opinions and knowledge from clinicians and other health providers in order to work on these problematic issues and question the status quo (Watson et al., 2016). To my mind, here would be an excellent example of how independent investigators with more diverse expertise might obtain more focused and useful recommendations if they collaborated with clinicians. The sensitivity of RCAs is highly salient in this regard, and there are many legal restrictions on the documentation that occurs in RCA panels. Finally, it is fair to say that RCA is reactive. By contrast, Hazard Analysis, just one method of assessing risks, seeks to analyse how failures occur in systems (Ericson, 2015). It has been successfully applied in the aviation industry, identifying the probability of an event occurring and the consequent degree of severity likely. I'm not qualified to discuss this topic in any detail. I mention it here for others to consider how such a proactive approach to patient safety and error could help reduce the ever-increasing number of sentinel events in the health sector.

So, from an LSP perspective, what do the sentinel events that I've described above have in common? For the Hong Kong events, we deliberately concentrated on specific types of communication failure, successfully linking them to the larger context of intergroup health communication in hospitals. Miscommunication also played a major role in Ryan Saunders' case, with busy health professionals not being as vigilant as they should have been – as stated in the coroner's report – and a lack of voice on the part of junior clinicians and nurses. There, the hospital hierarchy's inaction failed to ensure patient safety. Dr Jayant Patel's litany of sentinel events demonstrated a terrible situation that encompassed the acceptance by some of poor clinical skills, the power dynamics of a system ensuring that complaints were ignored, the fateful lack of checks and inquiries, and, not least, the blatant incompetence of Dr Patel himself. An LSP perspective allows us to review the circumstances with an intergroup lens, in turn helping us understand the motivations and cognitions of the key figures in these tragic events, all of which clearly demonstrate communication failure.

Open Disclosure

One final topic, intimately connected with RCA investigations, needs a mention, albeit rather briefly. Open disclosure is another part of dealing with sentinel events. This is a very sensitive and litigious area. Gallagher et al. (2007) wrote a review article on the issues of disclosing medical errors, and their comments are still as relevant today. Thomas Gallagher is an acknowledged expert in medical disclosure with numerous papers published over some 20 years. His work with other researchers continues (Olazo et al., 2023). As I showed in my discussion of sentinel events, health providers make mistakes; they are human and as susceptible to making errors as anyone. I doubt this could be contested. But the ramifications of such healthcare mistakes being made public cannot be ignored. Gallagher's (2007) paper identified key barriers to open disclosure of error. It stated that: "Historically physicians have been conflicted about disclosure. They have wanted to be open with patients but have been fearful of litigation, embarrassed, or unsure of effective disclosure strategies. A professional ethos of discretion or even coverup after harmful errors predominated, …" (Gallagher et al., 2007, p. 2713). It was clear from the report on Dr Patel that a code of silence prevented admission of his mistakes by fellow colleagues. We also saw that reporting a person as unfit to practice is not straightforward; others have their own agendas, which obscure transparency and preclude necessary action.

In the mid-2000s I worked at a metropolitan hospital in Australia, examining how health professionals managed their conversations with patients and/or families of patients who had experienced a serious sentinel event. The hospital was rolling out a training intervention to educate health professionals in best practice, specifically concerning how they discussed medical errors that had occurred. The aim of the intervention program was to train health professionals to manage the distress of both the patient and themselves. It's important to realise that most health professionals involved in or responsible for a sentinel event are devastated and face a number of personal and institutional challenges. What the program taught health professionals was how best to talk with highly distressed patients and their families. The program was ambitious and innovative, open to all personnel working in public health hospitals in Queensland. It was also highly skills-based, but, as you might by now expect, it did not introduce any theoretical framework to assist the health providers in their communication tasks. Any reference to intergroup dynamics was missing.

I know this chapter has covered a great deal of ground, and that much has been couched as rather negative. However, in this way, questions have arisen that I believe are essential for introducing novel ways of managing the wicked problem of healthcare and patient safety. These questions are equally relevant to earlier chapters:

1. How do the systems and institutional norms facilitate or hinder effective healthcare?
2. How can we effectively address healthcare miscommunication, sentinel events and the rigid hierarchical culture?
3. Who can assist in solving these problems?

Is it really all negative in healthcare? No, I don't believe it is, but successes and good news stories don't make the headlines very often. It's the sensational bad events that are picked up by the media. Health professionals are obliged to make official reports of any medical errors and cases of inadvertent patient harm. These cases are logged into the system and dealt with accordingly. Health professionals are not required to report on procedures that are successes. When good outcomes happen, the personnel concerned may often get no more than a pat on the back from work colleagues. Even so, health professionals can walk away from such good outcomes with a feeling of satisfaction about themselves and those with whom they work. While this is not peculiar to healthcare, it's also true that healthcare does attract a great deal of criticism and negative feedback. There would seem to be a marked imbalance between the celebration of successes and the public dissemination of bad outcomes. Thus, my observation on positive events in hospitals is that they should not be allowed to pass unnoticed. Rather, I would argue that a shift in focus to positivity may indeed be one way to start making changes for the better. In my own research over the past 10 years, I have always included questions to health professionals about the good events they have experienced and examples of good communication they can provide. I know from their narratives that good communication and strong collaboration do take place, and I will return to this theme of positivity in Chapter 8. So yes, this chapter may have seemed negative and bleak, but bear with me so that we may smile more in Chapter 8.

One last point I would like to make is that near misses are not investigated or understood enough. When something nearly goes wrong but is corrected, it represents a wonderful learning opportunity. How was the problem picked up? Who picked it up and when? How or why did one or more persons see that there was a problem? If we do not examine patient harm that nearly happened but didn't, we miss a golden opportunity to improve patient safety. Stucky et al. (2024) make the point that near misses occur more often than sentinel events and so are more invisible. Their paper is a call to encourage more critical thinking and to open up dialogue so that risk is reduced. Stucky and colleagues note that this kind of critical detective work can spotlight where weaknesses in the system, in teamwork, and in communication are occurring. Again, it is a proactive approach, and one that, it seems to me, requires more attention in healthcare than it's currently given.

My next chapter is shorter, being an introduction to how research is actually conducted: what do we have to bear in mind when we ask a research question, design a study and carry out that study?

Some Personal Review Points

This chapter has covered some negative aspects of healthcare, so let's begin our reflections on a positive note.

- When have you observed good healthcare outcomes that reflected effective communication? What made the communication effective and why?
- Do you believe the hospital culture influences communication between health professionals? If yes, why, and if no, why not?
- Think about a communication experience that you've had that was negative for you, for your work, for the patient or all three. What were the events that led up to the negative experience, and how was it resolved, if indeed it was?
- Have you ever been involved in a situation that caused patient harm? If yes, how much were you involved in the process of finding out what happened, and what were your impressions of the process?
- Do you believe healthcare represents a wicked problem? Why? – or why not?

Methodological Approaches to Studying Healthcare Communication

A colleague of mine was discussing some data that she had collected involving nurses. Her task had been to collect survey data from them before and after a particular training intervention. One of her aims was to find out if they rated their satisfaction in the workplace more highly after the intervention than before. The nurses rated satisfaction on a five-point numeric scale where 1 was "very dissatisfied" and 5 was "very satisfied". They were also asked to comment on why they had chosen their particular level of satisfaction. When the data were analysed, the researchers found that the nurses' satisfaction ratings had not increased. At first, they were disappointed because this suggested that the intervention had been unsuccessful. Numbers do not lie. However, they didn't have to rely solely on the satisfaction ratings; they could also read the nurses' written comments. These revealed new insights into what the nurses were experiencing. The researchers found that the intervention most likely had been successful, but that the nurses were now dissatisfied with another aspect of their work. If the researchers had collected only the rating scores, they would have missed this fact. Collecting different kinds of data to look at a specific question can give us more information than relying simply on numbers. Obtaining people's views tells us so much more.

I've often told this story to my students to show them the value of collecting more than one type of data to answer a research question. In this chapter, I'll describe the various types of data that can be collected and the different ways it can be analysed. Those of you who are communication scholars will already be familiar with most of what I'll cover. Health professionals who may not know how to design research should find, I hope, that this chapter will fill some gaps in their knowledge.

Research Process

There are many ways to carry out research, but I don't intend to cover every possible approach here. Instead, I'll focus on the way I conduct research, and I'll provide other readings for those who want to learn about alternative approaches.

From my perspective, having a research question that makes clear what you want to investigate is paramount. A focused question will dictate precisely what data need to be collected and analysed. For example, I may be interested in: "How much do patients participate in medical consultations?" This is a clear question, but there is yet a further important issue to consider. As a researcher, I must decide whether I am interested in collecting information about the patients' own perceptions of their participation: i.e., did they believe they participated a great deal or very little, or in collecting information about their actual participation behaviour: i.e., how much did they really participate in the consultations? Both approaches will provide an answer to the question, but they require different research methods.

To obtain a measure of patients' perceptions, the researcher needs to tap into what the patients thought about their capability for communicating during the medical encounter. Their level of participation is the "domain" (i.e., topic) of interest for the researcher. One way to obtain this information is by asking patients to complete a questionnaire containing a number of items (i.e., questions on different aspects of the encounter). Each item is measured by a scale that reflects perceptions of their level of participation, ranging from, say, 1 being "low participation" to 5 being "high participation". Because perceptions cannot be directly observed, the domain of interest is referred to as a "construct", something abstract rather than something concrete. The total score of their responses will provide a rating for the construct participation as perceived by the patients. Another way to achieve this same goal is to ask the patient some open-ended questions about how much they felt able to engage in the consultation. Patients would respond by writing or speaking about their perceptions of the interaction experienced. This second method provides more detailed information as it represents more than just numbers on a scale. The two approaches are termed quantitative and qualitative, respectively; I'll discuss them in more detail later in this chapter.

While the patients' own perceptions about their level of participation are important, these do not inform the researcher about how much they really did participate. Of course, this may not matter if perceptions are the researcher's desired construct. But on the other hand, if the researcher wants to know about the patients' actual behaviour, the interaction will have to be observed, and the behaviour recorded. Some researchers might want to investigate both the patients' perceptions of participation and their actual participation in order to assess the degree of concordance or discordance between the two. Why any differences might occur between them would be of interest. The answers could provide insights for health professionals, allowing them to consider how to better negotiate their future patient consultations.

Different Approaches to Methodology – Early and More Recent Work

Crafting research questions that address a construct, collecting appropriate data, and choosing the right methods of analysis are all critical aspects of methodology. Over thirty years ago, Street proposed that one solution to the problem of measuring interactions was to use multiple measures of behaviour and outcomes (Street Jr, 1993; Street, 1992). He suggested using measures of behaviour derived from both participants (insiders) and observers (outsiders), as well as quantitative and qualitative techniques (discussed a little further on), to better understand what the collected data might mean. As we've seen above, when both insider and outsider perspectives are obtained, the former provides insights into what participants were thinking when they performed a particular behaviour, and the latter provides an independent assessment from someone else about how that behaviour was assessed.

Early studies have provided ample evidence to show that participants' and observers' evaluations can differ markedly (e.g., Street, 1985; Street et al., 1988; Street & Wiemann, 1988). For example, Street et al. (1988) examined differences between participants' and observers' evaluations of forty social conversations, each between two students. The study focused on four specific speech behaviours: "speech rate, turn duration, interruptive speakovers, and vocal back-channels" (p. 339) . (Vocal back-channels represent momentary periods of often simultaneous speech, when the listener provides brief feedback either by monosyllabic responses such as "mhm" or "yeh", or by short phrases such as "I see".) They used three different presentational mediums (audio-visual, audio only, and transcript) apportioned among 240 undergraduate observers. By reference to the four speech behaviours, participants and observers were asked to evaluate five aspects of speakers' contributions, including communication satisfaction and communicative competence. Street and colleagues found that on all five aspects participants gave higher ratings to their partners than did the audio-visual and audio-only observers. In turn, audio-visual and audio-only observers gave higher ratings than transcript readers. However, there were many inconsistencies in the choice of speech behaviours to substantiate these ratings. Street et al., concluded that all participants, audio-visual and audio observers, and transcript readers not only varied in their evaluations of the same speakers, but also appeared to rely on different speech behaviours as evidence.

In another study, Street and Wiemann (1988) studied three aspects of the communication style of doctors: interpersonal involvement, communicative dominance (i.e., control) and expressiveness. They found that patients' perceptions of these differed significantly from the doctors' self-perceptions. In addition, these perceptual differences varied as a function of patient age and education. Patients over 50 years of age perceived doctors as more involved, less expressive and less dominant than did the doctors. In the 30–50-year age group, patients' perceptions and doctors' self-perceptions were fairly similar. Patients under 30 years also generally agreed with the doctors' self-perceptions, apart from the level of interpersonal involvement. In addition, less educated patients perceived doctors as less dominant than did the doctors themselves, and also less dominant than did the more educated patients. Street and Wiemann proposed that less educated patients tended to view doctors more favourably because of the latter's higher status. Interestingly, doctors' self-perceptions of communicative style were not related to patients' satisfaction with medical care. In conclusion, they argued that more attention should be focused on the verbal and non-verbal behaviours that created impressions of interpersonal involvement, dominance and expressiveness, and on the reasons for doctors' and patients' discrepant perceptions. They recommended that future research should attend to both participants in an interaction, which of course is a key principle of CAT.

More recently, Chevalier et al. (2020) employed both insider (patient and pharmacist) and outsider (observer) perspectives to data collected from hospital in-patients about to be discharged. They applied CAT strategies to explore the extent to which patients and pharmacists held similar perceptions concerning their shared interaction. While there was agreement on some aspects across all three raters (i.e., the patients, the pharmacists and the observer), there were also important discrepancies. For example, the pharmacists rated their ability to encourage patient responsibility for their healthcare lower than did either the patients or observer, while the observer rated the pharmacists lower for emotional expression than did the pharmacists themselves. Chevalier et al. noted that studies in communication are in their infancy in pharmacy, but the results support previous findings that the behaviour an individual believes they are performing successfully is not necessarily viewed as successful by outsiders.

The technique of using written passages is long established in health communication studies and was noted by Vanderford et al. (1997) as a powerful tool for understanding patients' perceptions. Brent Ruben asked participants to recall and describe their most memorable experience from the time they had been hospital inpatients (Ruben, 1990, 1993). Responses were classified into six thematic categories. The category most often reported was "personal treatment/caregiver interpersonal communication" (46.7%); the category "quality/quantity of information provided" accounted for only 5.8% of the data. The latter result may at first seem surprising, as Cegala and colleagues have placed great emphasis on information giving as a key task in an interaction (Cegala et al., 1996). However, Ruben's work supported the observations of Street and Wiemann (1987) that interpersonal communication is a critical factor in creating rapport between health provider and patient. The importance of experiencing accommodative emotional expression from their health provider was also shown by Watson and Gallois to be a vital predictor for patients reporting a positive health consultation (Watson & Gallois, 1999; Watson et al., 2012). These findings have been replicated many times and explain why information giving by the health provider may sometimes seem less important to the patient (Baker et al., 2021).

Quantitative and Qualitative Data Analysis

Quantitative researchers demonstrate the accuracy of their findings by determining their statistical significance. Statistical significance implies objective truth, not a result obtained by pure chance. But to this end, it is imperative that the questions (the items) that make up a set are both valid and reliable, requirements that we must now expand upon.

Validity

Validity is about truth and accuracy, ensuring that a questionnaire and its associated scale really measure the construct. Types of validity include content validity, face validity, criterion validity and construct validity. How can the researcher be sure that the topic of interest (the construct) is being captured accurately? First, the researcher must ensure that they have content validity. Does the set of questions reflect the relevant material? For example, if a survey is developed to ask nurses about how well nurse shift handovers are conducted, it's essential that germane questions are developed. Often, experts in the particular area are brought in to judge whether the proposed questions accurately cover the important issues and to ensure that irrelevant material is not included.

Face validity addresses whether the items look relevant and appear to tap into the construct. For example, if a study is being conducted on sun exposure and the use of sunscreen, participants would expect items relating to their behaviour when out in the sun. Participants taking the test should perceive relevance in the questions they are being asked. In reality, the researchers' questions may also include other factors concerning sun exposure, e.g., cultural or social norms in a particular locality, and how these might influence sun exposure behaviour. It's important that the participants believe the items to be relevant to the topic. If they don't, they may not take the survey seriously, and this would render the data obtained less meaningful.

Criterion validity concerns the comparison of data in a test to an earlier measure of the same construct. The variable is the specific subject of an item (each question or statement) that is capable of being measured or quantified by its associated scale. We would expect a high degree of similarity between the new data and the earlier measure. For example, participants' scores on a newly developed test should correlate closely with their scores on a similar test already validated. If the scores on the old test do not adequately predict the participants' scores on the new test, then the criterion validity is compromised.

Construct validity concerns ensuring that the construct has been appropriately investigated and that the test is actually capable of measuring it. The researcher must therefore clearly identify the relevant components that make up the construct. If the construct is mathematical ability, variables that should be associated with that construct need to correlate; variables that are not related (e.g., verbal ability) should not correlate. All relationships between variables and the construct must be tested.

Reliability

Reliability is a separate but equally important matter. It refers to the consistency of a score over time. For example, if I weigh myself each morning before breakfast, my bathroom scales should display a similar weight. If they show a widely differing weight every day, they are most likely not reliable. In statistics, it is essential to ensure that any scale devised to measure a construct, such as say, a sense of well-being, is reliable. The items making up the scale must also correlate in their measurements to an acceptably close degree with each other.

A calculation known as Cronbach's Alpha is used to ascertain how well all items in a set correlate (Cronbach, 1951). It is a measure of the internal consistency of a scale, an index of test reliability, and normally its calculation should produce a final figure of 0.70 or above. If a set of items had a Cronbach's Alpha of only 0.60, it might be that one particular item was not well correlated with the others. Removing that one item would improve overall reliability. Well-analysed quantitative statistics are meaningless if the items measured are not reliable. Remember too that you can create a scale that is highly reliable, but if it does not actually measure the construct, then it is not valid and therefore also meaningless. See the bibliography for more on this topic.

Further Research Considerations

However, ensuring that the items and scale are valid and reliable is only one part of data collection. The data must also be rigorous, and the findings must directly address the research. A significant outcome does not necessarily equate to a meaningful outcome. There are number of issues to consider. Crucially, we must ask whether a difference is shown to be statistically significant (i.e., not a random or chance occurrence), or actually meaningful (i.e., of actual importance)? For instance, clinical trials of drugs to reduce blood pressure will use statistical significance testing to analyse the results. Researchers will be looking for a significant effect. With a large sample of participants, small effects may actually be statistically significant due to the sample size. However, a reduction of between 5 and 10 in blood OBP[4] will be clinically meaningful. See Aitken et al. (2018).

Some researchers view qualitative research as being less rigorous than quantitative. However, although achieving rigour when analysing qualitative data is painstaking, when done correctly, it is extremely valuable for understanding the topic of interest. The onus is on the qualitative researcher to ensure their methodology is irreproachably rigorous and therefore open to scrutiny. They must convince us that their qualitative data are not chosen just to tell the story that suits them. Waitzkin (1990) highlighted the need to be vigilant against personal bias in qualitative analysis. Using his own earlier data, he argued for researchers to be aware of biases that might lead them to choose certain texts above others equally representative.

He set out eight criteria for analysing qualitative material to address issues of selectivity and bias: (1) use a representative sampling technique, (2) tape primary texts, (3) apply standardised coding rules to texts, (4) have more than one person prepare transcripts for analysis, (5) decide on rules of interpretation prior to examination of a text, (6) incorporate inter-rater reliability procedures to validate findings, (7) provide a summary of texts when findings are published and (8) present readers with the variability found in the texts. These guidelines, with the exception of the word "tape", which would nowadays be replaced by "record", still hold true today.

Regardless of whether the researcher is analysing quantitative or qualitative data, there are important stages to be completed before the actual collection of

---

[4] A blood pressure reading taken in a clinical setting.

data is undertaken. As we saw at the beginning of this chapter, the researcher must first establish their principal focus of interest. Only when this focus is clear can an appropriate study be designed. If data are collected before knowing precisely the questions being asked, it is very likely that the study will fall short in terms of meaningful outcomes. Knowing the focus of interest will lead to the second stage: identifying variables that are important for answering a research question. The third stage is to decide what kind of data should be collected. Whole books have been written on the subsequent analysis techniques, and the bibliography at the end of this chapter may prove useful for those who wish to pursue this topic further. Most researchers have a preferred data analysis approach. Typically, their research interests dictate whether they use quantitative or qualitative data analysis. We've now seen that each has its own merits and that some researchers will apply mixed methods, so combining these types of analysis. Using more than one dataset, e.g., one quantitative and one qualitative, is termed "data triangulation". It enhances the veracity of the findings (Noble & Heale, 2019).

Real-life Issues in Health Communication Data Collection

In reality, health communication researchers are often faced with the fact that the only data they can gather are participants' perceptions. My own recent research highlights this predicament. I've been working with colleagues at an emergency department in a public hospital. Our initial intention was to observe clinical handovers across different time shifts over a number of days. We were interested in observing specific communication behaviours that might occur during handover, such as the number of questions raised, who asked them and the different types of interruption. The highly sensitive nature of the hospital environment meant that the hospital Ethics Committee would not allow researchers on-site to observe handover. Instead, we had to settle for a survey with set questions, some of which were open-ended, thus allowing participants to write at length about their experiences. The survey thus provided us with the views of hospital emergency department staff, though this had not been our original intention.

Our questions covered different aspects, such as whether the time of the handover made a difference to its perceived quality, and whether a different handover leader changed the way it was conducted. Clearly, the responses would be the perceptions of the participants, and some people might question the veracity of their views. However, as I've shown earlier, perceptions do matter. If we were to find that different staff had differing perceptions about the efficiency of the clinical handover, then this would be an important finding. At the time of going to press, initial findings suggest that nurses and doctors do differ in their perceptions. Ideally, we would like to conduct observations and see for ourselves as outsiders what actually takes place. Making sense of why some staff perceive aspects of handover as occurring differently from other staff members could be taken into account, and reasons for the discrepancies might then become clearer. These two methods, survey and observation, represent an example of data triangulation. We remain hopeful that, at some point, observations will be allowed by the Ethics Committee.

Acknowledging Different Research Perspectives

Health communication researchers need to share their expertise with one another. By so doing, they will come to appreciate different approaches to the problems of studying this area. Why is this important? As noted in earlier chapters (especially Chapters 4 and 6), health communication research is interdisciplinary: there is great diversity in how health academics collect and analyse their data. Each discipline tends to have its own epistemological approach that directs how a topic is analysed and interpreted. These varying approaches involve the use of many techniques to address what are essentially often the same questions, though expressed in different ways. LSP researchers are interested in individuals' motivations, their levels of affect, and the cognitions that drive their talk. They try to understand the psychological processes that drive the communication. By contrast, for example, a conversation analysis (CA) researcher would never attempt to interpret what speakers might be feeling. They would examine the sequence of turns in a conversation in order to demonstrate how it is constructed or explore the patterns of words that speakers choose as they engage in the interaction. An LSP and a CA researcher might both examine the same text, but though they would be asking completely different questions, the answers might well be complementary.

Examining health communication research from different perspectives would allow a wider understanding of the health domain than is possible if researchers stick solely to their own methodologies. Such understanding has the potential not only to positively inform health communication but also to open up knowledge by researchers from different disciplines who generally do not read one another's work. The fact that academics often live in their own disciplinary silos leads to their research findings being presented in disparate media, not shared across the wider body of health communication academics. Academic journals that may welcome CA approaches may not accept papers that go beyond analysing word sequencing by incorporating psychological phenomena. In an ideal world, health communication researchers would ensure they were aware of other research outside of their own field; they would make efforts to explore what and how studies were being conducted by these different disciplines. By so doing, researchers could source other parts of the health communication process.

Recognising that there are different ways to address a particular research question and seeing the value in working with academics from different disciplines would give a researcher the potential to open doors for collaboration. In turn, such collaboration would encourage a broader readership of different health communication journals. Nowadays, researchers are being urged to work in teams. If the team included different disciplines and different methodological approaches, then the results of the research could offer a more macro perspective on the topic of interest.

In my own research, I have tried to connect with other disciplines beyond my own social psychology background. An eclectic approach is often adopted when the researcher investigates health communication as an intergroup phenomenon. In this chapter, I've covered some of these techniques and approaches. For more detailed and extensive information on methodology, see the suggested readings at the end of this chapter. However, whatever a researcher's methodological approach, there are key elements of research that hold true. If research is conducted with thoroughness and integrity, the findings will likely have relevance for all interested parties. Respecting the work of others who do not hold the same epistemological principles is the first step to understanding how others investigate the world of health communication.

New Wave of Research in the Late Twentieth and Early Twenty-first century

Finally, it is instructive to see how new software has radically expanded the way data are analysed. There are now many products on the market. An early example was NVivo, which provided qualitative researchers with software that made coding different types of text easier than it had been previously. Since its beginnings, it has moved from being a simple coding system to one that allows for sophisticated qualitative data analysis. For those interested, I recommend you visit: <https://lumivero.com/products/nvivo/>. Another software tool is Linguistic Inquiry and Word Count (LIWC), pronounced Luke. You can obtain information from their website: <https://www.liwc.app/>. I am familiar with two particular data mining software tools, which I'll briefly mention here. They provide interesting ways of analysing data.

Leximancer

Leximancer was developed in the 1990s as a text mining software tool. It can investigate reports, novels or interviews. Leximancer uses word association to create concepts from the input text. In this context, a concept is a list of words that frequently occur together and rarely occur apart. The analysis is designed in this way, as words that occur together (usually within a fixed two-sentence space) are often related to one another and reflect a fundamental idea. Co-occurrence statistics is used to create the concepts, which are independent of any researcher bias because they are formed from the actual text patterns. A number of concepts can represent a theme. If the data are interview texts, the speaker of the words may be identified. See the website for more information: <www.leximancer.com>.

A study that colleagues and I conducted concerned health professionals' views on clinical handover (Watson et al., 2014). The data included transcripts of interviews with doctors, nurses and allied health professionals. We found that time was a key issue for all health professionals. However, Leximancer also identified issues around time that were unique to each profession. The findings gave insights into issues that arose because of the ways that handover is managed at the hospital system's level. Importantly, the researcher can allow the data to emerge from the text without much interference. Changes that are imposed on the data are clearly listed, such as the omission of some words that would not be relevant.

Discursis

Discursis is another software tool developed at the University of Queensland. For a comprehensive visual review of Discursis, see Chevalier et al., (2018). From a transcript, Discursis creates a visual plot representing the chronological pattern of exchanges. By using different shapes and colours, this visual depiction can provide researchers with information about how well the interactants are engaging with each other. Each speaker's turn in a conversation is represented by concepts (i.e., groups of related words) that summarise the content of their speech. Across a conversation it can reveal how much the speakers are sharing similar concepts. Chevalier et al. (2018) analysed what CAT strategies were found in the interactions between patients and pharmacists. Discursis plots provided a visual map of the extent to which speakers were engaging in similar topics with each other. See: <www.atap.edu.au>.

Review

My aim in this chapter has been to provide you with a flavour of how research is generally conducted and how I conduct my own research. It was not intended as a comprehensive guide to qualitative and quantitative research methods. That said, I did think that to omit some mention of how LSP and other researchers conduct their endeavours left a bit of a gap in the story, and so I have provided a bibliography for the interested reader. Chapter 8 takes stock of what I've covered in this book, and there I offer suggestions for future directions in health communication research.

Some Personal Review Points

There may be many research questions you would like to ask, and there will be different ways you could answer them. Finding the right research question is not always straightforward. I've chosen just one research question, and I'd like you to consider different ways in which it could be answered. There is no right or wrong approach, as long as the research method you choose does try to answer the question.

You are interested in researching an aspect of clinical handover in your hospital. There are many questions you could ask, but you choose the following:

- How effective are bedside handovers compared to handovers away from the bedside?
- How did you define "effective" handover? You must be clear, so think about this carefully.

Further Reading

Maggetti, M., Gilardi, F., & Radaelli, C. (2013). *Designing research in the social sciences*. <https://doi.org/10.4135/9781473957664>

Whaley, B. B. (Ed.). (2014). *Research methods in health communication: Principles and application*. Routledge.

Future Directions

CAT has shown its value in exploring and explaining communication failure. The next step is to extend CAT as a vehicle for reducing communication failure in the health context. CAT has the potential to introduce a new pedagogy to communication accommodation competence training for health professionals, allowing new understanding for health professionals and patients about the complex system within which they communicate. (Watson et al., 2016, p. 164).

My colleagues and I wrote this in 2016. I want to expand now on how we can move forward by using CAT with an LSP approach.

I've covered a number of topics in this book. The choices I've made about what to include were driven by my goal to promote an LSP approach to the study of health communication. I hope I've provided researchers and health practitioners alike with relevant and helpful information about intergroup theory, so that they may gain insights into health communication behaviour. However, I've not suggested the LSP perspective as the only right way to conduct research, but, on the contrary, have taken a more inclusive approach.

We need interdisciplinary research to tackle the problems that health professionals and patients face in the current healthcare system. In this chapter, I want to enter into a dialogue with you and suggest some directions that will enable health communication research to move further forward. I use the word dialogue deliberately because I believe academics and health professionals who read this book can consider carefully what I am saying and create responses to my points. The desired outcome would be that these responses produce new ways of managing such communication. Academics can bring their interdisciplinary research skills to the table, and health professionals can contribute their knowledge and experience of how it really operates. Such a collaboration opens up exciting and innovative avenues for research and progress. The future directions I discuss here are complementary to LSP research. They could be adopted by researchers who do not normally apply an intergroup perspective to health communication. Diversity and thinking "outside the box" can facilitate change in this research area, whatever theoretical framework is applied. If we can collaborate and combine theories in a health context rather than depend on just one approach, we can expand our understanding of the complexities that exist.

One of the topics I now want to cover is the role CAT can play as an educational tool in health communication training interventions. Applying CAT in this way is very close to my heart because it means theory can translate into action and make a genuine difference. In Chapter 4, I made the observation that some researchers "want to obtain data without any real consideration of how health professionals and their patients may actually profit from any findings" (p. 51). They are naturally pleased to find significant results that support their theoretical frameworks, but they too often test the same theory again simply to demonstrate the same findings. I believe that researchers should use theory not only to predict and explain a certain phenomenon but also to work out how that phenomenon can be altered and improved. For me, knowledge gleaned should serve to make a practical difference. My own experience reflects this belief. After conducting a number of studies to test the presence of an intergroup culture in healthcare, it became clear to my colleagues and to me that not only was this extremely prevalent but that it impacted negatively on health communication. It also became apparent that we were no longer trying to demonstrate its existence; this we had done. Rather, we now needed to see how we could use this information to improve communication. This was and still remains the challenge. The application of CAT as an educational tool has great potential to make a significant difference.

Following this discussion of CAT as an educational tool, I'm going to introduce the application of another psychological theory that I was involved in while working in Hong Kong: "positive psychology". This approach reframes problems by addressing what is working well rather than what is going wrong; it is an important perspective that is too often overlooked. In Chapter 4, I mentioned the approach "to consult, to advocate and to use activism" (p. 51). Such an approach to improving healthcare requires engagement and commitment from both researchers and health professionals. Following this section, I will touch on the topic of leadership and its role in the health setting. I will not try to cover the whole of the leadership literature – it's a massive topic, and I am by no means a leadership expert. Rather, I will focus on the work of others who are more knowledgeable and who can illustrate aspects of leadership that, from my experience, are important. Finally, I'll discuss online medical consultations, which are becoming increasingly common post-COVID-19.

CAT as an Educational Tool

CAT has emerged over the last few years as a valuable educational tool in the healthcare context. It is a direction that I encourage new researchers to consider seriously and to develop. Again, I stress it should not be a stand-alone educational tool; it should form part of a package of approaches. Its particular contribution is its emphasis on the psychology of human actions as reflected in communication behaviour. I'll give some excellent examples of training intervention development, but much more is definitely needed. See also Giles and Jin (2025) for how CAT can be applied in such interventions for nurses.

The most recent work in the application of CAT is in research conducted by Dr Melanie Barlow for her doctoral dissertation. Previously a senior nurse in intensive care units (ICUs), Melanie discusses her work in more detail in the final chapter of this book, where she explains the value of an intergroup approach in addressing the particular problem in team communication of what is generally called "speaking up". This refers to a team member voicing a concern about patient safety. I believe her development of CAT in this context is dynamic and will have popular appeal for a wide range of researchers and health professionals. Rather than taking the traditional approach in health research, which is to focus on the sender of a message, Melanie has approached the problem of speaking up from the perspective of the receiver (M. Barlow, B. Watson, L. Jones, et al., 2023).

The value and contribution of her work in using CAT has expanded beyond health and attracted the attention of the aviation industry. Recently, Melanie, other colleagues and I have co-authored a book chapter on intergroup communication that applies Melanie's newly developed model of speaking up to communication on the flight deck (Barlow et al., 2025). Some of the co-authors are aviation experts who see its potential value to flightdeck interactions. The content of our aviation chapter is particularly pleasing to me because, for so long, healthcare has been leaning heavily on the aviation industry to improve patient safety. It's now time for healthcare to inform aviation about safety communication. This indeed represents a future direction beyond the health context.

Another practitioner and health provider who has developed CAT as a training tool is Dr Bernadette Chevalier. Her research has already been mentioned in Chapters 3 and 7. In Chapter 9 she offers her own insights into the value of an intergroup approach to research. As a practising pharmacist, she had frequently observed communication failures between other pharmacists and patients. While working at the University of Queensland, she developed an undergraduate training program, choosing CAT as the most appropriate educational tool to explore the communication issues she had regularly witnessed (Chevalier, Watson, & Cottrell, 2020). The program was designed for pharmacy students in their final year of university, before they went on to undertake internships in the workplace. It comprised three tutorials that addressed specific learning strategies and included pharmacist-patient role-play, which the students themselves then assessed. In addition, they completed a survey at three different time points: prior to the first tutorial, after completion of the three tutorials, and one year later when they were then interns employed in a pharmacy workplace (either a community pharmacy or a hospital pharmacy). The findings from Bernadette's longitudinal study demonstrate that learning CAT strategies can influence pharmacy students' subsequent communication behaviours for the better.

A third researcher who embarked on using CAT as an educational tool is Dr Rachyl Pines. While working as a volunteer at an emergency department hospital in the United States, she saw many examples of violence perpetrated by patients in the workplace. She decided to make this her doctoral thesis topic by investigating how CAT could assist in reducing such violent exchanges between patients and staff. I was fortunate to be one of her PhD advisors along with Professors Howard Giles and Karen Myers. She devised a training intervention study for 155 professionals representing a broad range of professions, including medical assistants, nurse practitioners and administrative personnel, all working for an organisation with seven different clinic locations (Pines et al., 2021). Prior to the training session, Rachyl held informal conversations with staff at the clinics about their experiences of workplace violence. This information was invaluable for the development of the training program because it made the scenarios that she designed authentic. These informal conversations also represented collaboration with frontline health professionals, demonstrating how important it is to learn what actually happens in an emergency department from the personnel involved.

At the training session, participants initially completed a survey about their knowledge of using communication strategies with aggressive patients. Next, they took part in simulations with volunteers who role-played aggressive patients, after which Rachyl provided an educational session explaining CAT strategies. Then followed a second round of simulations with volunteers again role-playing aggressive patients. Three months later, participants completed a follow-up survey. The longer-term outcome from this training intervention was positive. It showed enormous potential for assisting health professionals in managing and defusing workplace violence by applying these strategies with potentially aggressive patients. It was most heartening to see positive communication changes still in place after three months, especially as the training session itself had lasted for only about one hour.

These three examples of adopting CAT as an education intervention tool are really encouraging, and I am fortunate to have had some involvement with them. They go beyond giving health providers communication skills in that they examine what might be going on for each speaker in terms of motivation, cognitions, and goals. We can never know what a person is thinking or feeling; we can be aware only of their behaviour. However, recognising the need for such awareness and realising that we can't make assumptions about a specific behaviour and its cause is crucial. It means that the health provider can be more objective rather than simply judgemental, and this in turn can make a pivotal difference to how a conversation progresses.

Unfortunately, we cannot expect one training session always to produce miraculous results in communication. An early example of using CAT to educate health professionals was the work of Kristine Williams (2006). She designed a CAT training intervention program with the goal of improving communication between staff and residents at three nursing homes. Immediately following the intervention, staff were less patronising, less controlling, and demonstrated more respect for residents. When staff were reassessed two months later, findings suggested that the previous behaviours of exercising control and demonstrating little respect had returned. However, staff had not returned to their previous levels of patronising talk. While this finding was largely disappointing, it still demonstrates some encouraging behavioural changes. The message here is that one intervention session is not sufficient; it is important that refresher sessions and follow-up workshops are provided. The stresses and strains of working in the hospital context lead all too easily to deterioration in communication, even for those individuals with the best of intentions. Commitment to such additional interventions needs advocates whose mission must be to improve communication continually between health providers and patients.

I began Chapter 2 with a short anecdote from a workshop that Dr David Hewett and I conducted with different undergraduate health professional students. In these workshops, we introduced notions of tribal warfare existing between professions, and of CAT's philosophy and strategies. We showed the students some scenarios from the popular TV show "ER" that demonstrated issues around hospital hierarchy and culture. It was our distinct impression that the students resonated with the content. Regrettably, funding for the program ceased, and there has been no further progress as yet in developing a CAT educational tool for health professionals. Given the success of Melanie Barlow, Bernadette Chevalier and Rachyl Pines in pursuing their longitudinal studies, bringing the theory to both undergraduate students and to health professionals in hospitals would, I believe, be an important step forward in the improvement of communication between professions.

I want to make one last comment before I leave the educational aspect of CAT; it concerns how communication as a topic is often presented to students who decide to go into the health professions. Some years ago, I attended a talk by Professor Srikant Sarangi, Director of the Centre for Discourse and Practice at the Danish Institute of Humanities and Medicine. He made the point that teachers of student health professionals often refer to two types of skill that students must learn. Hard skills are specific technical skills that must be acquired for professional competency. Soft skills are more general transferable skills, used for instance in communication and relationship management. Referring to communication as a soft rather than a hard skill can lead students unthinkingly to consider it easily acquired and therefore far less important.

Communication is not a soft skill. It requires dedication to understand how to communicate with someone about their particular situation. For instance, every person's reaction to a diagnosis is unique. Whatever their theoretical stance, communication researchers must not perpetuate the myth of a soft skill. The evidence for the complexities of miscommunication demonstrates that it is anything but a soft skill. Similarly, in our recent chapter on flightdeck communication, Melanie Barlow and I made the point that using the term non-technical to describe communication skills is equally dismissive and usually leads to a loss of audience attention at the very outset of any lecture on the topic (Barlow et al., 2025). Effective and responsible communication is hard work: it takes training and practice.

Positive Psychology

I now turn to the theory of positive psychology (developed by Martin Seligman and others), which I believe could add great value to health communication research. It isn't my intention to give an in-depth account of the theory, but rather to provide an overview and demonstrate why it has such value. While I had been aware of the positive psychology approach, I did not use it until I developed a course in Hong Kong. It was then that I realised how its application had the potential to improve mental health and resilience throughout one's life. Christopher Peterson summed up the essence of positive psychology when he said it is "the scientific study of what goes right in life" (Peterson & Castro, 2006, p. 4). I refer you here to Martin Seligman's book "Flourish" (Seligman, 2011), in which he provides a history of its development – it's a great starting point for those interested. Peterson and Castro (2006) noted that Seligman introduced the term "positive psychology" while President of the American Psychological Association. His rationale for this new term was his belief that there had been too much emphasis on pathology, and although this had led to great advances in treating some mental health disorders, it had come at a high cost. That cost was in ignoring the strengths that individuals possess. Seligman proposed that it was time to redress the balance by focusing equally on strengths and weaknesses. See: <https://www.ted.com/talks/martin_seligman_the_new_era_of_positive_psychology/transcript?subtitle=en>.

In his talk, Seligman noted that interventions were traditionally designed to focus on an individual's problems and deficiencies. He argued that "positive psychology" recognised explicitly that psychology should be concerned with strengths as much as weaknesses, helping individuals build the best in their lives as well as repairing the worst. It should be concerned with making people's lives fulfilling and with nurturing talent, as much as with healing illness. There is much more to positive psychology, but one important take-home message is especially relevant here. Positive psychology is about achieving a sense of well-being; it is not about seeking to be happy. Pursuit of pleasure or happiness rarely makes people happy. I leave it to you to investigate further.

Positive psychology focuses on ensuring individuals recognise their strengths and use these to assist them with weaknesses. Such a focus helps individuals develop resilience. There is also an emerging body of research that places "positive communication" as critical to health and well-being. The Routledge Handbook of Positive Communication (Editors: Muñiz-Velázquez & Pulido, 2018) incorporates research into how communication in many different areas influences how we communicate and interact with others. I see strong connections between CAT and the study of positive communication. Some of my future work will be concerned with marrying CAT and positive communication in healthcare. See also my bibliography at the end of this chapter.

I am certain that a shift in focus to positivity is one way of making changes for the better. In my own research over the past 10 years, I have always included questions for health professionals about the good events they have experienced and any examples of good communication they can provide. Indeed, if I approached a hospital board about research that sought to examine only what goes wrong, I know they would show me the door. Instead, I say that I want to look at what goes well in health communication and to discover how that comes about. I know from the narratives that health professionals have related to me that good communication and strong collaboration do exist.

Finding out what goes well and what works well will undoubtedly inform us about how to do things better. Yes, we do learn from mistakes and near misses (Stucky et al., 2024), but we can also learn so much from positive events. Why must we always focus on the negative? As a researcher, I have experienced a situation where two separate departments within a hospital were in stark contrast. In one, there was constant infighting between doctors, nurses, and other staff, yet in the other was collegiality, teamwork and an atmosphere of trust and good humour. How does this happen? Why not unpack what is happening in the exemplary department in order to inform the dysfunctional one? But attention is always given to conflict and error with a directive to "sort it out". How much more rewarding for all if we examine good teamwork and good leadership and see these as examples that other departments and hospitals can profit from. Applying principles of positive psychology to the health context will provide much more information to help improve patient safety and allow us to move away from focusing only on failure and sentinel events. Of course, miscommunication must be carefully investigated, but striking a balance between positive and negative communication is an important step forward.

Consult– Advocate – Action!

I want to revisit these three action points because, alongside CAT as an educational tool and the application of positive psychology, researchers need to be alert and sensitive. I want to reinforce the point that they be receptive to what health professionals say they need. I'm not suggesting that they blindly follow only what health professionals suggest, though as frontline operators their input clearly matters. It may well be that professionals don't see alternatives to how they routinely work. Social scientists and academics in other disciplines can offer new ideas for changing behaviours that are outside the health providers' experience. Such discussions require respectful consultations that engage everyone. Researchers should not simply push for research that gets them published, important though that is. They must also consider how their research can translate into improving hospital staff communication and patient outcomes.

Taking a consultative approach will, in most cases, assist the researcher in finding an advocate within the healthcare context who will support and promote their topic. Having someone on the inside of an organisation means that there is at least one champion who will try to ensure research is completed and, where necessary, continued to a second phase. After 30 years of running research projects in Australia and Hong Kong, I know first-hand that such a person is pure gold. Of course, having more than one advocate is a bonus, but in my experience, research cannot succeed without at least one person in a position to promote the program. A researcher needs to consider very carefully who is best placed to be an advocate. Senior management or department heads are certainly in positions that give them some clout for pushing ideas forward. But by now it will come as no surprise to you to learn that doctors are particularly invaluable as advocates.

Consultation brings advocates, and as I have indicated, this creates a state of activism. Activism will generate change. Because of the inherently wicked problem of health miscommunication, the researcher, their team and the advocates must all be vigilant in looking for unexpected outcomes. These outcomes may be positive, but they can also be negative. The latter instance does not necessarily mean that the research has failed, but rather that an evaluation stage and an investigation are required. Once again, it will take more than one discipline working on the problems to generate new ways to manage and negotiate research with health professionals. For a meaningful outcome, there should be a working committee made up of the researchers and all appropriate levels of health provider, which can examine the research progress. As you can imagine, this takes massive commitment from all involved. Getting such commitment requires ongoing consultation and connections with advocates so that activism may naturally follow.

Leadership

I now turn to the role of leadership. As I said at the outset of this chapter, leadership is a large area of research which I cannot possibly cover here. I want to highlight research that has examined the leadership field by applying intergroup theory. I'll then discuss what I have learned about leadership problems in the health context. I should also clarify that when I talk about leaders, I am referring to anyone who manages a team, is in a senior leadership role, or is the leader of an organisation. Leadership occurs at all levels of responsibility. As you read this section, I would like you to think about how much you may play a role as a leader in whatever capacity.

I first refer to a paper written by Hogg et al. (2012). Michael Hogg and colleagues drew on social identity theory (SIT) to discuss issues around leadership. I particularly like this paper because the authors include a health context scenario to discuss leadership in an intergroup context. They make the point that group membership is an important part of human social engagement. To this end, as we have seen, individuals seek to identify with their ingroup members and distinguish themselves from outgroups. It is not difficult to envisage that if a leader is a representative of one particular outgroup, they may not be readily welcomed by those who identify with other groups. Hogg et al. (2012) state that what is needed is a dedicated theory of intergroup leadership in order to explain and negotiate leadership challenges of this nature.

It will come as no surprise that I am supportive of leadership research that adopts an intergroup perspective, not because it is the "right" way to understand what might enhance leadership skills, but because Hogg and his colleagues approach leadership in a way that resonates with my own experiences in the health setting. Hogg et al. (2012) suggest that for leadership to be successful in situations that are strongly intergroup and where conflict exists, the leader must create an *intergroup relational identity*. The first step to achieving this is to recognise that intergroup relations exist. In the past, it was assumed that individuals would work better together if they all subscribed to some superordinate identity. For example, all employees would be expected to identify with their particular organisation first and foremost. In the hospital setting, this identification might be with the actual hospital site. The assumption was that if everyone were to identify as being employees of the hospital, they would all relate to one another and accordingly work well together. However, as noted by Hogg: "Attempts to encourage superordinate re-categorisation can be viewed as an identity threat that is resisted, often fiercely" (Hogg, 2016 p. 8).

To explain why encouraging a superordinate identity that overrides other sub-group identities doesn't actually hold up, I will give an example from the health setting. A doctor trains for many years to become first a junior doctor in a hospital, and later a specialist in their chosen field. As I noted in Chapter 4, doctors identify with their specialty as a distinct group that sets them apart from other specialties. After so much time and dedication devoted to achieving their professional identity, it is highly important to them. It is also true that at times they may see identification with a particular hospital as salient. For example, it may be important for a doctor to promote and advertise their own hospital when they meet doctors from other locations. But overall, their sense of belonging is linked more to their profession. Doctors may be asked to become part of a multidisciplinary team, which I noted in Chapter 4 as happening more and more with advances in medicine. However, encouraging doctors to see themselves as team members rather than simply as doctors with expertise is potentially a threat to their professional identity. Clearly, they are perfectly capable of being good team players while still identifying with their specialty. But learning to be a good team player is a separate issue, albeit related, and goes back to how doctors are trained in their undergraduate years.

The 2012 paper by Hogg and colleagues emphasised leadership and intergroup relational identity, in essence stating that intergroup relations must be acknowledged. The leader must be someone who connects the different groups and encourages intergroup collaboration. They must make explicit the importance of each group (e.g., doctors, nurses, allied health professionals, administrative personnel) and how the hospital is made up of all these sub-groups. Each hospital sub-group brings its own unique and significant contribution to patient care; the hospital itself cannot exist without them. In his 2015 paper, Hogg further stated that a leader should be a persuasive speaker whose message "should explain how the whole is significantly greater than the parts and depends on the distinctive and valued qualities that each group brings to the table; it should identify the intergroup collaborative relationship as a unique way to arrive at outcomes closely associated with group identity but not threatening to perceived group distinctiveness and value" (Hogg, 2015, p. 194).

My colleagues and I conducted research at a US hospital that had introduced dyadic leadership. Teams of two (or occasionally three, i.e., triads) worked together as co-leaders. The aim of these teams was to bring together the management of various aspects in order to ensure improvements. One non-clinical senior leader observed of these teams that:

"You have the physician leader handling a lot of physician-related clinical issues; you have your nurse leader who really kind of – the quality, the safety, and you have your business leader. And when you've got those three, kind of your three-legged stool, working – it's a pretty powerful thing" (Leach et al., 2021, p. 366). This study neatly exemplifies the notion of relational identity and the value of recognising the relevance of sub-groups in the hospital.

There are, of course, other important aspects of leadership that I don't cover fully here. Kelly and Hearld (2020) reviewed literature in the health context, examining the connection between leadership style and staff burnout. They noted the important role that leaders can play, and that while leadership style matters, goal setting and task allocation are also key factors for leaders in reducing such burnout. On a related topic, Specchia et al. (2021) conducted a systematic review of leadership styles and nurse job satisfaction. Their findings reinforced the fact that leadership style was correlated with nurse satisfaction, showing that some forms of leadership had a more negative effect than others. What these papers and those of others demonstrate is that leadership needs to be learned (see the bibliography for further reading). Some people may be natural leaders, but the skills and psychological principles that underpin leadership behaviour require some form of training.

At this juncture, I want to discuss briefly my own observations about leadership and, where relevant, refer to my previous research with colleagues. It's been my experience that in many hospitals, there is no training for staff who gravitate from being frontline carers to managers and leaders. As I've shown in the previous section, this is a serious problem that requires more attention. If healthcare communication is to improve, then the calibre of leaders must also be enhanced. I say this as a result of the many conversations I have had with various levels and types of clinician.

Some years ago, my colleagues and I conducted a study in Australia and the United States (Leach et al., 2021). We wrote about clinical managers and made the point that "good leaders made the difference to the healthcare quality and patient safety" (p. 361). This was irrespective of whether they worked in the United States or Australia. In the same study, and again across both countries, frontline clinicians who did not have management roles reported that senior clinical managers and leaders showed little understanding of what frontline clinicians needed and had expectations that were unrealistic in terms of patient care. This last comment reflects the observation by Kelly and Hearld (2020) that different leadership styles can directly impact the extent to which staff in healthcare experience burnout.

At a large metropolitan hospital in Brisbane, I conducted some research involving interviews with a diverse range of staff. One of the members of the executive board observed: "One of the things is [*sic*] that is changing is that clinicians now have to become managers and their management skills are not all they might be. Some are excellent, some are ordinary and some are awful" (Jones et al., 2008 p.308). Regrettably, I don't see anything changing as we move into 2026. Management and leadership training is still often lacking in hospitals. Recent research outlines some of the problems clinicians face when in leadership roles (Imran et al., 2021). It is a fact that in order to be promoted, health providers must take on these senior roles, but if they are not equipped for them or not suited to them, problems will inevitably arise.

It is apparent that different professions have different requirements of their leaders. In the same way that doctors, nurses and allied health professionals were all concerned about time in the handover study I described in Chapter 4, so too do they have different leadership needs. In research not published at the time of going to press, Ivy Wu and I spoke to doctors, nurses and allied health professionals about what they thought made a good leader. Leadership for these three groups was a very important influence on their ability to deliver quality patient care. Nurses, and to some extent allied health professionals, reported on the specific tasks within their own fields that leaders should focus upon. Both professions emphasised that leaders should proactively back staff who might need support and guidance. Doctors also acknowledged these qualities for a leader, but they also identified intangible tasks that leaders must manage effectively.

For example, doctors stated that a leader must be able to understand the bigger picture of the hospital system and its particular facilities for appropriate coordination of patient care.

According to all three groups we interviewed, the key attributes for a good leader consisted of being a good role model for their staff, being proactive across different contexts, and having the ability to manage conflictual situations. They also emphasised that leaders should have attained a high level of ability in their particular profession and be excellent communicators. And finally they reported that ensuring the right people with the right experience became leaders was paramount to the foundations of a cohesive work environment. This would allow staff to develop their levels of competency and collaborative ability. The message that came across from these participants was that leadership skills must be taught and that not everyone has the capacity to lead. Often, staff are put into leadership roles when they are better suited to supporting a leader. Better training and evaluation of potentially strong leaders would be a first step in establishing more effective leadership.

We need to look to researchers across different disciplines to work out what needs to be prioritised in order to ensure healthy leadership becomes a part of healthcare. I say this because, patently, it is currently lacking. Effective leadership matters in order to ensure staff well-being, patient safety and the investigation of sentinel events. Bringing an intergroup perspective to this research is but one critical element.

Online Medical Consultations

Online medical consultations are becoming increasingly commonplace. They will be important for new directions in communication research. Throughout this book, I've focused on areas of research with which I've been heavily involved, not ones with which I have had less connection. However, recently I've taken part in some research into this developing field and so can relate my own experiences as well as observations from the literature.

A few years ago, I was associated with research investigating the effectiveness of online consultations. Some of the problems concerned the actual technology. Poor internet connections and time lapses, resulting in a person's face freezing on-screen, sometimes interfered with effective consultations. Over time, these frustrating problems have become less frequent, but nonetheless they still occur, and health providers need to be prepared for these mishaps. However, putting those technical and software issues to one side, we must recognise that online communication is a different medium with its own characteristics. A key issue in early research on visual online consultation concerned the direction of gaze for each speaker. When talking to a person, it really matters that you are actually looking at them. Thus, checking the accuracy of the camera angle becomes critical. It's also important that each speaker, if they can be seen, looks attentive and is actively engaged with the other speaker. I have often observed participants in online meetings being distracted and clearly disengaging themselves from the ongoing conversation. Individuals sometimes forget that they can be seen looking at something else.

The COVID-19 pandemic demanded a change from face-to-face to online medical consultations. After COVID-19, online medical consultations remain very common and nowadays are sometimes the preferred medium of communication. White et al. (2024) noted that there was little advice for health professionals on how to achieve effective online consultations. In my early work, I have also observed this gap. The aim of White and colleagues was to develop evidence-based resources that could be used for online consultations. In their in-depth study, they recorded online consultations, surveyed patients, and interviewed GPs and patients. Their findings highlighted that a doctor's communication style was critical to the success of such consultations. They, of course, did not apply CAT, and so had their own terms for what was an effective communication style. However, their findings align with CAT in that appropriate interpretability, discourse management, interpersonal control and emotional expression are all critical features in ensuring an effective consultation.

Another study that did not specifically invoke CAT but did take an LSP approach was one I supervised with a Master's student, Nova Li, in Hong Kong. Her research into online consultations in China, was conducted at the time of COVID-19 (Li et al., 2025). Her findings reveal some important aspects that will require further exploration. Many of her participant patients preferred online consultations because they did not have to travel to see the doctor; it was a faster process than face-to-face, and they found it generally more efficient. However, there were two important caveats. Firstly, the participants themselves recognised that in some cases they did need to see the doctor physically, and that an online consultation was therefore insufficient. Secondly, they reported that emotional care was often missing from their online consultations. This was especially the case when the consultations were text-only. The study demonstrated that patients wanted the health provider to actively show care that is both interpersonal and empathic. Thus, emphasis should be given in training doctors to be more patient-centred during online consultations.

From the studies reported here, I see a real opportunity for CAT to inform health providers about how they should communicate virtually. It's clear to me, and I'm sure to many LSP researchers, that CAT should now be used to research online medical consultations. The findings from these studies could then be employed to train health professionals in applying theory to these.

Review

In this chapter, I have proposed ways in which the topics in Chapters 2–6 could be expanded. My emphasis has been on an LSP approach and using CAT as a powerful educational tool in health settings. I have also suggested bringing positive psychology into play. This would allow a celebration of the successes in healthcare, of which there are many, but which regrettably are too frequently overshadowed by more negative effects. Such an approach would assist in discovering how near misses occur and what prevents them from becoming sentinel events. Knowing what strengths exist and recognising weaknesses is an educational blend to provide more knowledge on how to get things right more often. I've reiterated the importance of health researchers connecting with health providers so that the latter can be included in research programs. This engagement would assist with locating advocates and lead to appropriate action. I've also introduced the role of leadership, a feature that seems to be seriously lacking in some aspects of healthcare. If with hindsight we now revisit the case of Dr Patel in Chapter 6, we can see how the presence of effective, strong and transparent leadership emphasising intergroup relational identities might well have prevented the tragic events that unfolded. And finally, I've touched on the emerging importance of online consultations as another area that requires research using an LSP perspective.

In the final chapter, I have asked colleagues who are or have been clinicians to give their thoughts on why an intergroup perspective is such an important part of health communication research. I also share the experiences of a close friend of mine who underwent a serious trauma, spending over a year in a spinal unit.

Some Personal Review Points

Below are some topics for you to reflect upon. I also think that the breadth of this chapter will have given you an opportunity to devise your own review points.

- Can you see how CAT could work in your work environment to enhance relationships between individuals? If yes, what would you focus on? If no, why not?
- I have argued that communication in some contexts can be difficult and uncomfortable, even though it is often described as a "soft skill" or a "non-technical"

skill. Raising awareness that communication can be a challenge is important. Do you agree with this last statement? If yes, why, and if no, why not?

- From your experience, would a culture that actively recognises successful patient outcomes rather than focusing only on bad outcomes make any difference to your own working environment? Can you explain your view on this?
- What is a good leader to you? How much importance do you give to communication in their role?

Further Reading

Haslam, S. A., Reicher, S. D., & Platow, M. J. (2011). *The new psychology of leadership: Identity, influence and power* (1 ed.). Psychology Press. <https://doi.org/10.4324/9780203833896>

Mickel, A. E. (2024). Positive communication practices for enhancing collaboration. *International Journal of Business Communication*, *61*(4), 876–902. <https://doi.org/10.1177/23294884241263552>

Socha, T., & Pitts, M. J. (2012). *The positive side of interpersonal communication*. Peter Lang Verlag. <https://www.peterlang.com/document/1143803>

The oxford handbook of positive psychology. (2021). Oxford University Press. <https://doi.org/10.1093/oxfordhb/9780199396511.001.0001>

What do Health Providers and a Patient Say About Health Communication?

In this final chapter, three health providers, all colleagues of mine, share their views on the value of including an intergroup perspective in health communication research. When I asked them if they would be willing to contribute to this book, I deliberately didn't prompt them to cover any specific issues. I asked them simply to discuss from their own experience what they have found to be important in healthcare communication. I am thrilled that all three colleagues agreed to accept my invitation. I very much value their knowledge and experience, and because they come from different health professions, they will each bring their own unique perspective to this chapter. I also confirmed that any edits to their contributions (e.g., typos) would be kept to an absolute minimum. How they each voice their opinion matters just as much as what they say.

Following their contributions, and to complete the picture, I asked a close friend of mine if I might interview her and write up her personal story so as to obtain her insights as a patient. I have known Julie for over 40 years. In 2021, she had a fall which left her quadriplegic. Julie's subsequent dependence on health providers offers a thought-provoking insight into how communication exchanges between them and her can enhance or reduce a patient's quality of life in the hospital setting. David, Bernadette, and Melanie tell their story in their own words. Julie related her story to me in a recorded interview. I then wrote it up, but I can confirm that Julie subsequently read the account and agreed that it represented exactly what she had experienced.

Understanding Health Communication from an Intergroup Perspective by Dr David G. Hewett, MBBS, MSc, PhD and FRACP Associate Professor and Gastroenterologist

David is a gastroenterologist at Colonoscopy Clinic in Brisbane, and also a health services researcher at The University of Queensland in Australia. He has worked in public and private health systems in Australia and the United States. His clinical interests include colorectal cancer screening, familial cancer and polyposis syndromes, and the technical performance of colonoscopy; he has published widely on new colonoscopic techniques, technologies and methods of training. His research interests include quality of patient care, intergroup communication and relations between clinicians, and medical education.

David's Narrative

> A woman with kidney failure and recurrent severe gastrointestinal bleeding was admitted to hospital; this was her fourth admission in three weeks, with no cause yet found for her bleeding. This time, she was admitted to the care of the internal medicine department, but her bleeding required coordination by the gastroenterology department. Tension between these departments and conflict about who was responsible led to long delays in her care. The patient stayed in hospital for four days with no further treatment, despite increasingly explicit pleas for help with her care from internal medicine. The internal medicine doctors devised a strategy to force the involvement of gastroenterology, by sending her home from hospital and refusing further involvement in her care. This plan was put into her medical record and communicated to the emergency department. She was discharged but was readmitted the next day with catastrophic gastrointestinal bleeding that required emergency surgery. She died shortly afterwards in the intensive care unit (from Hewett et al., 2013, who provide a discourse analysis of the medical record).

This is a real-life story about a patient in a large Australian hospital. Hospitals like this are complex, socio-technical environments comprising vast numbers of individual health care providers. Early in my career as a physician and gastroenterologist, I observed (and participated in) similar episodes of conflict between hospital doctors. Doctors and all other health care providers are differentiated from each other through their membership of different groups, such as workgroups, teams, departments, specialties or professions. As a member of the gastroenterology department, I was required to collaborate and negotiate the care of patients with doctors and health professionals from other specialties, such as emergency medicine, surgery, intensive care, and anaesthesia. I knew of occasions where inter-specialty power play (such as in this example) compromised the care of patients and led to adverse outcomes.

Miscommunication has long been considered a leading cause of inadvertent patient harm and adverse events in hospitals. In response, communication skills training for health providers has adopted communication competence and human factors approaches that emphasise deficits in individual provider skills and promote checklists, structured communication tools and situational briefing models. However, these simplistic approaches, reflecting research at the interpersonal level, fail to acknowledge the social environment and system within which health providers are required to negotiate care. They do not consider the subtleties of communication and language, such as those used during inter-specialty power play in an intergroup context where power, status and competition are powerful drivers of interprofessional interaction.

As a participant and player in these inter-specialty turf wars, I knew that structured communication tools were not the answer to promoting high-quality, collaborative care between doctors. Miscommunication in health does not solely arise from skills deficits, nor does it involve perpetrators and victims. Like tribes or gangs, each health professional group has a distinct culture and identity, governed to some extent by explicit rules, but more importantly by unstated social norms and values. The specialty-based organisational structure of hospitals and health services encourages the development of a tribal or "intergroup climate", in which inter-specialty or interprofessional rivalry can occur. In this climate, issues relating to power, control, status and competition become relevant, and group memberships influence individual behaviour and communication. An intergroup lens explicitly acknowledges the highly hierarchical and role-based structures of the health system, in which status and professional categorisations or memberships are highly salient.

I embarked on a body of work examining communication between hospital doctors from an intergroup perspective, using a language and social psychology approach. We uncovered a climate of intergroup disharmony in which patient care is not the highest priority. Specialty identity and intergroup conflict are invoked over ambiguous and contested responsibilities for patient care. Patient care becomes a commodity over which identities are negotiated and conflict enacted, such that patients themselves become entangled in intergroup conflict.

These extracts from interviews with hospital specialists highlight the intergroup climate:

> It's difficult if you've admitted a patient under a General Medical unit to get the Gastros to consult, because they're not responsible for them ... if the patient was in under Gastro,

> they'd have a vested interest to do the scope, to get them out of hospital as soon as possible. If they're under someone else, that interest isn't so acute [General Medicine doctor].

> It becomes a bit of a tug of war. We have had issues where there's been reluctance to accept the patient ... [it's] very hard for us because then we're searching for the best approach to match the patient when you don't feel like you're getting support from other teams. You have competing interests and you're in the middle trying to make sure that the patient's going to get their follow up [Emergency Medicine doctor].

Health professionals have a strong sense of their disciplinary and professional memberships, which pervades interactions. Perceived differences in status and power between specialties can foster tensions and misunderstandings between doctors. Power play between specialties is particularly evident under conditions of workload pressures or resource shortages, such as often occurs in government-funded or "public" hospitals. Specialty departments are required to compete for scarce resources, and patients are caught in the conflict. Patient care becomes a tool used to negotiate and act out inter-specialty power play, such that threats to withhold care become a communicative tactic.

Rather than focusing on interpersonal communication competence and blaming personal and cultural deficiencies for miscommunication, the intergroup approach in fact highlights how communication can be used strategically, with sophisticated communication tactics used to negotiate care between professions and specialties. Both motivated communication failure and miscommunication are caused by intergroup conflict or rivalry.

An intergroup approach implicates the structural organisation of patient care in the genesis of an intergroup climate. Clinical work is a process of negotiation within a health system in which structural factors govern ownership of patients and the specialised skills and equipment required for their care. In the patient example above, we see the consequences of ambiguous and contested ownership of a patient promoting the expression of professional identity at the expense of an identity and values focused on patient care, with resulting negative consequences.

Although challenging for researchers and potentially confronting for health care providers, an intergroup approach is so important in healthcare to raise awareness of the miscommunication that occurs when identities and perverse motivations driven by identity get in the way of best practice. Explicating intergroup dynamics in this high-risk environment, where one in ten patients is inadvertently harmed by the care they receive, has the potential to change the face of health care and save lives. Hospitals and health services are intergroup organisations, and the quality of patient care must be addressed through intergroup means.

How a Social Psychology Approach with a Framework like CAT that Accounts for Group Identities Can Help Us Communicate Effectively within Our Complex Health Context by Dr Bernadette Chevalier, *BSc Pharm, ACPR, PhD*

Bernadette is teaching internationally trained pharmacists within the Faculty of Pharmacy and Pharmaceutical Science at the University of Alberta, Canada. She practised as a hospital pharmacist for more than 20 years: in general medicine as a resident, in neonatal intensive care and later as a drug utilisation pharmacist and pharmacist educator. Bernadette has also worked part-time as a community pharmacist at different points throughout her career. She completed an internship in multiple primary care clinics to become relicensed as a Canadian pharmacist after completing her PhD at the University of Queensland in Australia. Her main research interests and publication focus include pharmacy practice research, and communication between pharmacists and patients and with other health professionals.

Bernadette's Narrative

The SARS-CoV-2 pandemic has had a devastating effect globally, and in these post-pandemic years, many people continue to experience a great deal of uncertainty, frustration, fear and an overall world-weariness. Health professionals and the systems in which they work have been pushed to their limits and beyond. They face many systemic challenges in delivering quality health care in a time-poor working environment with severe staff shortages, as well as having to adapt to rapid changes and expanding practice roles put in place to compensate for the paucity of staff. Some patients and their families have, in turn, experienced delayed treatment, dissatisfaction with their healthcare interactions and negative health outcomes, leaving them angry, frustrated, frightened and distrustful of their care providers. Many systemic healthcare issues are beyond the control of individual health professionals. However, effective communication and the way in which they interact with patients, their families and with other health professionals are key in making a difference to patients' care. Empathetic conversations that reassure and empower patients, and respectful and supportive interactions with health professional colleagues, are needed now more than ever.

Using a psychosocial approach with a specific framework, such as CAT, to account for group identities, such as those of healthcare consumers, and the dynamics between individual health professions, can facilitate the understanding of interactions between health professionals and with patients within complex healthcare environments.

As a pharmacist for nearly 30 years and in an academic environment for 10, I have observed both stellar and cringeworthy examples of pharmacists' exchanges with patients and other health professionals. My own practice evolved from a provider-centric approach where I was focused on putting together clever care plans to share with the team. I enjoyed working within a team and a strong group identity emerged. My interactions with patients and caregivers were secondary at that time. As my life and health care experience grew, I became concerned about how pharmacists centred their practice on the "what" we did instead of "how" we did our roles. I overheard a conversation between two pharmacists in our shared clinical office area discussing with annoyance a patient's nonadherence, "Look I gave them the information- what more do they want? If they don't do what they're supposed to do – that's their problem!" In the same clinical office space, I have also listened to a different group of pharmacists having an empathetic conversation about a patient's chemotherapy treatment and their difficult life situation. This contrast between callousness and caring communication behaviours ignited my desire to study how well hospital pharmacists communicate with patients. I moved halfway around the world with my family to start a PhD at the University of Queensland with Bernadette Watson as one of my advisors. Very little research in hospital pharmacist communication had been conducted to date, and I enthusiastically began my academic career delving into CAT to understand what was happening in pharmacist-patient interactions.

In my research, I observed a range of CAT behaviours in 48 pharmacist-patient exchanges. One particular example of accommodative emotional expression behaviour between a pharmacist and a patient took place in an emergency room. Empathy and concern were clearly demonstrated by a pharmacist completing an admission medication review with a patient in severe respiratory distress. While going over the patient's chart, the pharmacist discovered a note about the patient having a dog at home. After inquiring about her dog, the patient relayed that the dog was at home and arrangements for feeding and care had not yet been made. Then the patient on oxygen broke down and began to cry. The pharmacist gently touched her hand, looked into her face and told her that she would contact the social worker to help make arrangements for her dog's care. The pharmacist made the call, the patient appeared reassured and a few more medication issues were addressed. The social worker arrived within 10 minutes, the pharmacist finished up and handed over to the social worker. The patient's nurse mouthed a "thank you" to the pharmacist on her way out. In these respectful and conscientious interactions between the pharmacist and other health professionals, the pharmacist utilised accommodative emotional expression, discourse management and interpersonal control strategies in engaging and communicating effectively in her handover to others.

All CAT strategies were applied by most study pharmacists, and interestingly, many combined communication behaviours such as reassurance (Emotional Expression), well-explained medication information (Interpretability) and rationale for treatment (Interpersonal Control). Sometimes these combinations appeared like an information-reassurance-information sandwich in which the pharmacist might review potential side effects, then reassure the patient with the low likelihood of experiencing them and follow this with more information about how to manage these should they occur. The addition of rationale into an information sandwich was often included to encourage adherence to therapy by having the patient understand how and why the medication was important to their therapy. The ability to effectively communicate and accommodate patients' conversational needs by the pharmacists in my research did not appear to be affected by their age, professional experience or gender, but was observed most often in those who reflected about their patient exchanges in our post-interaction interviews.

In my own clinical practice, in addition to the provision of appropriate written and verbal information, hearing patients' stories, reassuring upset or overwhelmed patients and encouraging them to be active participants in their own health care are my main CAT go-to behaviours. For example, more recently, while working as a community pharmacist, I had a conversation with a young single mother about her successful 18 months of opioid agonist treatment. I congratulated and validated her experience by saying, "That's amazing. It must have been very difficult - Good for you!" She became teary-eyed, thanked me, and said she really appreciated me saying so. For a vulnerable person like this young woman, the demonstration of these communication behaviours seemed to be impactful.

In terms of how I communicated and addressed my health professional colleagues, specifically physicians, I began to shift about midway in my career from referring to them as "Doctor so and so" to using their full name or first name only. For example, almost all physicians I worked with would sign off on their emails with their first name only. I would then reciprocate by addressing them only by their first name. For those that did not, I'd use their full name in an email, "Hi John Smith". When introducing students to the team, I would introduce them as "This is John/John Smith. He's one of the neonatologists in the unit". This practice predated my knowledge of CAT and my awareness of interpersonal communication behaviours that promote equality between speakers. I simply noticed that our relationships and interactions changed subtly to become more equitable when I did so. But now I have the theoretical background to support my decision.

In my current role/identity, I am a lecturer in a university bridging program for internationally trained pharmacists who are completing the multi-step process to become licensed as Canadian pharmacists. To help these learners successfully navigate the cultural differences and communication challenges in Canadian practice, I utilise most CAT strategies but emphasise three. The first is emotional expression (reassurance, showing/helping them how to be successful in the program and in practice). The second is interpretability (clear wording and communication as English is a second language for most learners). The third is interpersonal control. This last strategy promotes equality between patients and learners through shared decision making. Such decision making accounts for patient preferences, as many learners come from more authoritarian countries where power differentials are more evident. For my communication lectures, I have translated findings from my research to create a CAT-based communication assessment rubric which provides learners with explicit examples of expected communication behaviours. I have also adapted this rubric for pharmacists' conversations with other health professionals.

As health professionals, we live in uncertain times and work in challenging and stressful environments. Having effective conversations and making meaningful connections with patients and with our health professional colleagues may also grant us a reprieve from the difficulties of the outside world.

CAT as a Tool to Inform Health Professionals about Speaking up by Dr Melanie Barlow PhD, RN, MN, G. Cert Ed., SFHEA

Melanie is a registered nurse, specialising in intensive care. She has a long history of health education within hospitals and higher education. She currently works as Associate Professor at the Australian Catholic University as the national academic lead for the specialised learning environments and simulation training. Melanie has a passion for experiential learning and for using this methodology to support the learning and development of future health professionals, particularly in enhancing intra- and interprofessional communication to improve patient safety.

Melanie's Narrative

As a registered nurse with 30 years' experience, you could say that I have had a few professional communication interactions. Transitioning from a new graduate nurse working in medical/surgical inpatient wards, to cardiac and trauma intensive care units in Australia and the United Kingdom, you learn the hard way how to (somewhat) navigate conversations with different professions and hierarchy. During my clinical practice, I felt that how I spoke to my nursing colleagues day to day was not how I spoke to medical or allied health professionals, yet at the time I didn't really understand why that was, until one day, it all became horribly clear.

I had never been taught how to speak up (that came later), but I knew as a nurse and patient advocate, it was my professional responsibility to. So, on a shift in the trauma ICU when the most senior medical consultant stated my patient was ready to come off the ventilator, I realised I had a very different assessment of the situation. In front of the large multidisciplinary team, I knew in that moment I had to voice my concern. I naively thought, I am part of this team, and I have a point of view, surely this opinion is welcomed. I was mistaken. I was publicly put in my place and told not to question. Unfortunately, my assessment was correct, and it was the patient who felt the consequences of that poor intergroup interaction.

As an educator many years later, that interaction drove me to find a better way. I had been involved in designing and delivering vocational simulation-based interprofessional education for a number of years. In interprofessional education, the aim is for differing health professions to learn with, from and about each other. This is essential, as every health profession at an undergraduate level is taught and socialised within their own discipline. Therefore, each health profession produces graduates with unique ways of communicating and upon graduating, it is expected that they naturally know how to come together as a team. The differing communication styles directly influence conversational dynamics between health professions. Yet what interprofessional programs often espouse is equality amongst the professions; we "are all one team and all input is valued". Yes, important, and in some teams true. Overwhelmingly though, the lived reality of health professions on the clinical floor is that traditional health hierarchies still exist. Generally, medical officers sit higher in the hierarchical structure than nurses; junior nurses/medical officers have less of a voice than senior nurses/medical officers. Here is where interprofessional education needs to be informed by communication theory such as CAT, which recognises and tangibly accounts for these very real and ever-present intergroup dynamics. From my example alone it is clear that intergroup communication has clear and direct implications on patient safety.

Healthcare organisations teach people to speak up. That is, to voice or assert a concern to prevent error and harm. This emphasis to speak up is important as medical error is a leading cause of patient harm in health services (Douglas et al., 2021; World Health Organization, 2019a). Traditionally, speaking up programs tell clinicians what to say and how to say it via an assertiveness pathway to escalate their concern. This speaking up script is taught to be stated regardless of who it is the person is speaking to (profession or seniority level) and regardless of the context of the situation. Most programs will also say, "listen when someone speaks up", but fundamentally, these programs don't teach people how to effectively listen, how to manage their defensiveness if their decision is being challenged, nor how to respectfully respond. The focus is on the act of speaking up, fundamentally one side of a conversation. This was evident in my clinical example. Why? Because these conversations haven't been viewed through an intergroup lens, and until recently no evidence existed in the healthcare speaking up literature on how to train the receiver of speaking up messages. This is what I aimed to change through my research.

After six years and three empirical studies exploring and observing receiver behaviour in healthcare speaking up interactions, my findings showed:

1. Speaking up interactions are categorically intergroup in nature. Health profession and seniority level influence:
   - how the phrasing of speaking up messages is evaluated. Scripted assertiveness pathways are important for the speaker as they have been shown to help voice concerns (Hanson et al., 2020); however, my findings showed that these messages were received and evaluated differently according to profession (M. Barlow, B. Watson, E. Jones, et al., 2023; M. Barlow, B. Watson, L. Jones, et al., 2023). From the receiver's perspective, one size does not fit all. Different health disciplines evaluated the speaking up message differently depending on how the message was phrased and the speaker's perceived manner and tone of voice. Nurses, midwives and allied health professionals liked longer more relational messages, whereas medical officers tended to want short, sharp (typically evaluated as non-accommodative) messages (M. Barlow, B. Watson, E. Jones, et al., 2023).
   - if positive attributions are made or not of the speaker's intent. The making of positive attributions about the speaker was identified as a key enabler of more effective receivership and accommodative interactions (M. Barlow, B. Watson, L. Jones, et al., 2023).
2. Context is everything. Nurses/midwives did not like being spoken up to in the presence of other people (patient or health team members). It influenced how they heard and responded to the messages. Medical officer communication behaviour was not reported to be impeded by the presence of others (M. Barlow, B. Watson, L. Jones, et al., 2023). Currently, speaking up programs don't teach or account for context. This needs to be considered to enhance message reception and the quality of the safety conversations.
3. Speaking up does not just occur up the hierarchy. It occurs peer to peer and also frequently down the hierarchy. Being a junior clinician is really

difficult. Literature shows it is hard as a junior to speak up against hierarchy (Peadon et al., 2020) and my research shows that often juniors are also receivers of speaking-up messages occurring down the hierarchy. Regardless of how respectfully the message is delivered, being junior and being spoken up to caused strong emotional reactions and influenced communication behaviour, such as just following orders even if it may lead to harm (Barlow et al., 2024).

From the findings it is clear where we need to go to improve intergroup communication in order to help enhance patient safety.

- Health organisations need to stop focusing speaking up training on the **act** of speaking up, rather shift the focus to the speaking up **interaction**, teaching equally the speaker and receiver how to effectively negotiate patient safety concerns (Melanie Barlow et al., 2023).
- To do this requires understanding that each person, due to professional socialisation, knowledge and prior experiences, will perceive the same situation differently. Therefore, it is not about who is more correct, but rather what are the differing perspectives, and what is the right thing to do in this particular context and situation. To achieve this requires an ability to accommodatively negotiate and be communicatively adaptive.
- These training programs need to include validated communication theory that acknowledges and accounts for intergroup dynamics, such as CAT, to help provide tangible strategies on how to navigate the intergroup differences and to know how to adapt these strategies in differing situations.

Navigating intergroup dynamics is not innately easy, even for more experienced clinicians. To be honest, even for those, like me, who have created training programs to help enable more effective intergroup conversations. What does enable more effective intergroup dynamics is an awareness of what is driving our own behaviour and that of my conversational partner. Understanding the influence of social identity helps to attribute positive intent and positive regard to the other; it helps position us to be more curious rather than certain. What I advocate for the future is training programs that focus more on communication interactions where both speaker and receiver are equally accountable and trained. This will help shift the focus from purely advocating my stance to more accommodative negotiations, where perspectives are shared and resolutions achieved.

Response to these Three Contributions

David, Bernadette and Melanie, from their own practical experience, have described the intergroup environment in the healthcare system. Before I received their contributions, I was reflecting on how best I could respond to what they might have written. However, as I then read each piece, I saw that they mirrored precisely the comments that I have made throughout this book. They speak quite dramatically of the conflict between health professions, of the fact that patient care is often complex, of the ongoing problems with a hierarchical system and how all of these factors play out every day.

Their comments emphasise what a wicked problem miscommunication in healthcare represents. It has so many components, and these can so often be at odds with patient care. Health professionals face numerous pressures that exacerbate already existing intergroup conflict. Resource shortages, long hours and fatigue all factor in. Additionally, there are systemic issues over which healthcare providers have no control. They follow procedure, and as Julie's story below will show, that does not always assist with quality patient care.

All three contributors show how the adoption of an intergroup perspective brings awareness and better understanding of the ways in which the complex hierarchical hospital structure influences the goals that health providers possess for any one encounter. They feel a need to protect themselves within the hospital environment, and this attitude can impact negatively on quality patient care. What each contributor identifies is that an intergroup perspective provides a rubric not only for recognising why miscommunication occurs but also for furnishing a means to make communication effective. The psychological principles that underpin human behaviour as an intergroup phenomenon speak directly to improving health provider interactions. This can result only in an enhanced healthcare environment. I am truly grateful for the time they have taken to voice their opinions. Let us now turn our attention to Julie, so that we may hear her perspective as a recipient of healthcare in a hospital.

Julie's Story of Her Time in a Hospital Spinal Unit, as Related to Me

My friend Julie has spent 18 months in hospital. She had been a busy full-time project manager with many travel and business commitments, but overnight Julie was suddenly paralysed by a fall at home. In all the years that I have known her, she has always been a strong and resilient person. But her journey from a fall at home in 2021, first to an intensive care unit, then to a spinal unit for over a year, to living now in 2025 is nothing short of remarkable. Although totally paralysed and needing 24-hour care, Julie has mastered voice control computer technology, enabling her to return to her previous position as a project manager and to work full-time from home. In addition, she enjoys going to the theatre and ballet with friends, while her passion for cooking, albeit now by overseeing rather than participating physically, has not diminished.

Julie knew I was writing a book on health communication; I was very pleased when she accepted my invitation to be interviewed about her healthcare experiences. The difference between Julie's perspective and those of David, Bernadette, and Melanie is two-fold. Firstly, Julie is not a health professional; she is reporting her experiences as a patient. Secondly, Julie is not familiar with an intergroup perspective on communication. I was very careful, therefore, to ask her only very broad questions, allowing her to express what was important to her. Our recorded conversation lasted for half an hour.

I started by asking Julie about any positive aspects of her hospital stay. Julie recalled a nurse (we will call her "Susan") who cared for her in the spinal unit. She had been in the unit for 40 years, and Julie said she was down to earth, was a direct speaker and wasn't afraid to give you information she thought you needed to know. Susan explained the whys and wherefores of procedures and about what was happening or going to happen. She didn't just say that she needed to do such and such; she told Julie why she was doing it. This was really helpful. The impact of this kind of communication behaviour was that Julie felt that she was not just having things done to her; rather, she understood why they needed to be done. This was in contrast to how other doctors and nurses behaved, who never explained what they were doing but just did it. Julie attributed Susan's communication style to her long nursing experience. They had lots of conversations and got to know each other on a personal level as well as at the nurse-patient level. She was forthright, which Julie appreciated.

Another example of communication that made Julie feel more like an individual was her conversations with an older male nurse. He also got to know her well, and while plans were being made for Julie to return to her own home, he accompanied her in the ambulance to her home along with occupational therapists and others whose job it was to assess the progress being made on house modifications. On one of these short visits to her home, Julie gave him some plants from her garden. When it was time for Julie to leave the spinal unit and go home permanently, he gave her some seedlings from the plants she'd given him. His level of care was what she needed, and again, she appreciated him as a straight talker; their conversations recognised the individuality of each.

I asked Julie to sum up what good communication was for her. She readily admitted that everyone is different, but felt it was important for staff to learn that everyone needs a different style of communication. The health provider needs to recognise that what is palatable for one patient may not be sufficient for another. Should they sugarcoat the information or not? Julie was quick to point out that the staff were not bad, but that for a number of reasons they did not address her needs.

We then moved on to communication that had not worked well. She said that in the few months she was in the ICU, she did not get to know the nurses. For one thing there were so many of them and, as many patients were unconscious, talking to patients was not within their scope. Because Julie was in the ICU for longer than most patients, she was given a side room, the rationale being that at night she would have a quieter environment than in the main ICU ward. However, because so many of the patients were unconscious, the nursing staff tended not to lower their voices during the night shift, therefore keeping her awake. She said she learned more about their personal lives and their house renovations than she wanted to know. She was unable to talk at night because she has a tracheostomy. During the night the tracheostomy tube cuff was routinely inflated. This prevented air from passing between the vocal cords, thus rendering Julie unable to speak. She could therefore not tell the nurses to speak more quietly. She felt constantly sleep deprived.

Julie observed how the hospital system and its weighty administrative processes influenced patient care. She felt that there was a defined process for patients suffering a spinal cord injury, from the time a patient is admitted to the unit to their finally leaving. Having such a process sounded reasonable, but Julie observed that the process was kept a secret from patients. Health providers only drip-fed information. What Julie wanted and needed were some timelines. Even if these timelines were changed, that could be explained, but no one was willing to explain the reasons behind decisions. She knew that everyone's injury was unique to them, but she found that any kind of discussion about progress was not forthcoming. This was extremely frustrating. All she wanted was for the staff to explain the process to her as it affected her case. One example she gave occurred when they were trialling different wheelchairs for her. She was not involved in the discussions about which chair was chosen or why. While some people might not have been interested, Julie was. This was why she had got along so well with Susan. Julie summed it up by the fact that they did not tailor communication to the individual but rather followed due process without explanation, even when the patient required more details. They gave only bits of information for the current moment, but this spoon-feeding did not work for Julie.

While in the spinal unit Julie was assigned a psychologist. The first time the psychologist arrived, he came up to her bed in the open ward and said that he wanted to discuss her psychological well-being and any problems she was experiencing. Julie could not believe someone was giving her a counselling session in an open room. This made her extremely cross. She asked the psychologist if he would normally conduct private sessions in the waiting room of a clinic. He replied, "No" to which Julie responded, "Well why are you doing that here with me?" She wanted a private room as she did not want all the other patients to know about her personal business. The next time, he suggested having a session on the open balcony, maybe because he thought this might be preferred. But the balcony, which was adjacent to the spinal unit, had people coming and going all the time – it was anything but private. Eventually, after much hassle, a treatment room was provided, but then the psychologist was assigned another placement in a different part of the hospital. She never saw another psychologist.

Julie's time in the spinal unit occurred during the COVID-19 pandemic. Staff were stretched due to sickness, and there were also staff shortages. This was problematic for staff and patients. Julie was quick to note that the staff were doing the best they could, often in difficult circumstances. But as I was talking to Julie, it seemed to me that there were some very small changes that would make a big difference to patients. Julie said that she rarely saw doctors in the spinal unit. The doctors would come once a week, and the consultant did not have time for conversations with patients. The treatment plan was discussed, but because there was so much discussion about the chemical composition of the prescribed drugs and how they interacted, it was by definition not an inclusive conversation. As she said, "treatment was done to you". Communication wasn't so good, even though it was not deliberately bad. Treatment appeared to be like a factory process line.

As we were finishing our conversation, I asked Julie what else stood out to her during her time in the spinal unit. She said the hardest thing was being confined to a bed space 24/7. She could not leave the unit in her wheelchair without a ventilator nurse accompanying her. Officially, each patient on a ventilator is assigned their own one-on-one ventilator-trained nurse, but in reality, this did not happen. Without a dedicated ventilator nurse, no staff were available to get her away from her bed. Julie felt tethered and plugged into the wall. Because she could voice activate her iPad, and so could watch movies etc., she was deemed as "fine". At the very least, she would have loved to have been taken out onto the balcony, but this rarely happened. She said she felt isolated. Her bright points in the day were when visitors came; then she could go onto the balcony. She remarked that she could ask a nurse to carry out only one task at a time rather than saying she had a list of two or three things that needed doing. The nurses could not stay with a patient to carry out a list of jobs. Indeed, it was not uncommon for Julie to ask for something to be done, only to find that the nurse had been called off somewhere else. She again attributed this to a lack of resources and staff shortages.

Julie is now back home. I asked her to tell me what it is like for her now. She said that she now has more control, and her brilliant team of carers talk to her and listen to her. They sometimes ask for advice so that conversations are two-way and symbiotic. When Julie is able to go out to a restaurant, the carers attending her join in and share the meal. Similarly, they will also share the meals cooked at home if they fit with their dietary customs. The carers have told Julie that other clients don't share. Because of Julie's love of international cuisine, she wants her carers, who come from many different countries, to experience a wide range of different dishes. They are family. Recently, Julie went to the housewarming of one of them. I went as well, and we enjoyed superb Nepalese food.

Julie does still have to attend outpatient appointments but said that the communication is very perfunctory. This communication behaviour may again be due to time constraints and resources. She had two final stories to share. One concerned a time when she needed to have a new ventilator to replace her old one. She went to the hospital to get the accurate settings for the new ventilator that she was going to receive. She was told she would need to stay overnight for observation to ensure all was well. However, the overnight stay never transpired because the staff could not actually fit the new ventilator. Upon her arrival, they found that the new ventilator plug connection was not the right one. In addition, when the settings were checked, they were not right. She had to show the ventilator nurse how the new ventilator operated, as the nurse had not been trained to use this type of equipment. Julie was told that the consultant was not available and that she would have to wait for the on-call doctor to come and try to sort out the problem. She had already been at the hospital for some hours, and there was no clear indication of when the on-call doctor would appear, or indeed if he could assist. She said that she had had enough and wanted to go home. Up until very recently, Julie was still waiting for the new ventilator to be fitted and was still using the old one, but as she said, delays are common. With respect to this event, she said it seemed to be all about having policies and processes that weighed the staff down and did not work. For example, in exasperation Julie commented: "Why don't staff get trained on the new ventilator? What is the reasoning?"

Julie went back to the spinal unit recently to visit a patient to give peer support. She had been insistent that she and the patient would go across the road from the hospital for lunch. She arranged the time she would arrive. When Julie came to the spinal unit, no one had prepared the patient, and he was still in bed. It looked at first as though they would not be able to leave the unit. The staff suggested they could have coffee on the balcony. Julie flatly refused and said the patient needed to have a change of scenery. After waiting some time, they were able to go down to the coffee shop in the main hospital. This was better than nothing, as although it was not outside the hospital, it was away from the spinal unit. Following their conversation, Julie hoped she had given this person belief that he could have a life outside of the hospital.

Closing Comments on Julie's Story

Unlike my other three contributors, Julie has not studied the approach I take to health communication. My questions to her were very general and open-ended. However, important elements from CAT came through, as did other issues around the wicked problems in the hospital setting. Importantly, too, Julie recognised that no one was being deliberately unhelpful; sometimes the problem was due to a lack of awareness of her needs, and sometimes other constraints. This confirms my message that, along with communication failure, other factors exist. Staff shortages, poor resources and a bureaucracy with its own rules and regulations within the hospital's organisational structure all play a part. These are problems that need attention by a wide range of experts from different disciplines. Addressing these problems would also take commitment and serious collaborative consultation from many vested parties. Changes can take place if we alter the communication dynamics by applying an LSP approach. Julie's story highlighted not only the many difficulties she faced but also how some staff were able to improve her day-to-day experience.

Susan, the nurse, treated Julie as an individual. She assessed Julie and saw her as a woman who sought information about what was happening. It could be that at first, she tested Julie out by providing her with extra information; when Julie responded positively to this approach, she continued. This I do not know. For Julie, she made a big difference because of the way she interacted and cared for her. The same individuality was recognised by the older male nurse who took time to talk to her, reciprocating later with a gift of seedlings for her garden when she moved back home. What came across to me was that Julie wanted to be engaged with her treatment in whatever way she could, and not simply have things "done to her". A change in the way Julie had been spoken to would have made a difference, and her feelings of isolation and frustration could have been at the very least reduced. Seeing the patient as an individual and engaging them in communication that is two-way and empowering mattered very much to her. From my own experiences, both in my research and in my own personal life, being seen as more than a symptom when consulting a health provider changes the communication in a positive way. I also think it's important to note that Julie's present carers have admitted that not all their clients are as inclusive as Julie in sharing meals. This shows how patient preferences can shape the relationship and signify different patient needs.

Closing Comment on This Book

I have nearly reached the end of this book. At times, I have found the writing difficult, yet always rewarding. For those who think the issues in healthcare are too big and too wicked to fix, I have one short but telling anecdote I want to leave with you. Can any one of us make a difference by ourselves?

I believe this final story demonstrates an emphatic "yes". It concerns Julie's experience in trying to obtain a new ventilator. More recently she mentioned to me that she now has her new ventilator. At long last it had been successfully calibrated and fitted. She told me that in total, she had gone to the hospital five times before she got it correctly calibrated. Each visit, apart from the last one, had resulted in only more problems, discomfort and an unsuccessful outcome.

One of the main issues causing the problems was that when Julie stayed in the hospital overnight, the consultant was not there to oversee the process. She said that she was taking up a bed for someone who was ill and who really needed that bed. Julie was there for equipment maintenance; she was not an acute patient. She suggested to the consultant that it would be more efficient if she were offered a daytime appointment and took up a bed in the Sleep Clinic. She had noticed that during the day, the Sleep Clinic was unused. In addition, it would mean that the consultant and his team would be readily accessible. The use of this clinic for respiratory patients had never occurred to the hospital team. They were delighted and said they would put this procedure in place for future patients. Julie made a difference not only for herself, because the ventilator check went smoothly and she was able to go home in the afternoon, but also for a potential patient who would not be denied a hospital bed in the Acute Respiratory Ward. This is a win-win story. Julie's story gave me great hope for the future. Every individual can make a difference. It just requires perseverance and innovative thought. And it reflects a closing comment that I made in a talk at the University of California, Santa Barbara, in October 2019. His Holiness The Dalai Lama was purported to have once said:

> If you think you are too small to make a difference,
> think of the mosquito:

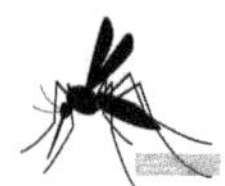

Bibliography

Abraham, J., Kannampallil, T., & Patel, V. L. (2014). A systematic review of the literature on the evaluation of handoff tools: Implications for research and practice [Journal Article]. *Journal of the American Medical Informatics Association*, *21*(1), 154–162. <https://doi.org/10.1136/amiajnl-2012-001351>

Aitken, C. G. G., Wilson, A., & Sleeman, R. (2018). Statistical significance—meaningful or not. *Law, Probability and Risk*, *17*(2), 157–162. <https://doi.org/10.1093/lpr/mgy005>

Al-Btoush, A., & El-Bcheraoui, C. (2024). Challenges affecting migrant healthcare workers while adjusting to new healthcare environments: A scoping review. *Human Resources for Health*, *22*(1), 56. <https://doi.org/10.1186/s12960-024-00941-w>

Al Shamsi, H., Almutairi, A. G., Al Mashrafi, S., & Al Kalbani, T. (2020). Implications of language barriers for healthcare: A systematic review. *Oman Medical Journal*, *35*(2), e122. <https://doi.org/10.5001/omj.2020.40>

Anderson, E. S., & Lennox, A. (2009). The Leicester model of interprofessional education: Developing, delivering and learning from student voices for 10 years. *Journal of Interprofessional Care*, *23*(6), 557–573. <https://doi.org/10.3109/13561820903051451>

Australian Commission on Safety and Quality in Health Care. (2012). *Safety and quality improvement guide standard 6: Clinical handover.*

Australian Commission on Safety and Quality in Health Care ACSQHC. (2020). *Australian sentinel event list (version 2): Specifications. Sydney: .*

Baker, D. W., Parker, R. M., Williams, M. V., Coates, W. C., & Pitkin, K. (1996). Use and effectiveness of interpreters in an emergency department. *JAMA*, *275*(10), 783–788. <https://doi.org/10.1001/jama.1996.03530340047028>

Baker, S. (2006, June). Willingness to communicate and participation in health interactions. International Conference of Language and Social Psychology, Bonn, Germany.

Baker, S. C., & MacIntyre, P. D. (2003). The role of gender and immersion in communication and second language orientations. *Language Learning*, *53*(S1), 65–96. <https://doi.org/10.1111/0023-8333.00224>

Baker, S. C., & Watson, B. M. (2015). How patients perceive their doctors' communication: Implications for patient willingness to communicate. *Journal of Language and Social Psychology*, *34*, 621–639 <https://doi.org/10.1177/0261927x15587015>

Baker, S. C., & Watson, B. M. (2020). Investigating the association between internet health information use and patient willingness to communicate with health care providers. *Health Communication*, *35*(6), 716–725. <https://doi.org/10.1080/10410236.2019.1584778>

Baker, S. C., & Watson, B. M. (2025). Balancing Good Medicine and Good Communication: Doctors' Perspectives on Health Consultations and How They Accommodate to Their Patients. *Health Communication*, 1–13. https://doi.org/10.1080/10410236.2025.2526024

Baker, S. C., Watson, B. M., Jamieson, B., & Jamieson, R. (2021). How do patients define satisfaction? The role of patient perceptions of their participation and health provider emotional expression. *Health Communication*, *36*(14), 1970–1979. <https://doi.org/10.1080/10410236.2020.1808409>

Baker, W. (2024). Intercultural communication. *ELT Journal*, *78*(2), 212–215. <https://doi.org/10.1093/elt/ccad040>

Bales, R. F. (1950). *Interaction process analysis; a method for the study of small groups*. Addison-Wesley.

Barlow, M. (2021). Enhancing intergroup communication in healthcare: The role of the receiver. *Focus on Health Professional Education: A Multi-Professional Journal*, *22*(3), 78–84. <https://doi.org/10.11157/fohpe.v22i3.523>

Barlow, M., Watson, B., Jones, E., Maccallum, F., & Morse, K. J. (2023). The influence of professional identity on how the receiver receives and responds to a speaking up message: A cross-sectional study. *BMC Nursing*, *22*(1), 26. <https://doi.org/10.1186/s12912-023-01178-z>

Barlow, M., Watson, B., Jones, E., Morse, C., & Maccallum, F. (2024). The application of communication accommodation theory to understand receiver reactions in healthcare speaking up interactions. *Journal of Interprofessional Care*, *38*(1), 42–51. <https://doi.org/10.1080/13561820.2023.2249939>

Barlow, M., Watson, B., Jones, L., Morse, K. J., Maccallum, F., & Rudolph, J. (2023). Building a workplace-based learning culture: The "receiver's" perspective on speaking up. *The Journal of Applied Behavioral Science*, *0*(0). <https://doi.org/10.1177/00218863231190951>

Barlow, M., Watson, B., Jones, L., Williams, C., & Mavin, T. (2025). Expanding cat beyond health to the aviation industry. . In H. Giles, D. Markowitz, & D. Clementson (Eds.), *New directions for, and panaceas arising from, communication accommodation theory*. Peter Lang.

Barlow, M., Watson, B., Morse, K., Jones, E., & Maccallum, F. (2023). React, reframe and engage. Establishing a receiver mindset for more effective safety negotiations. *Journal of Health Organization and Management*, *ahead-of-print*(ahead-of-print). <https://doi.org/10.1108/JHOM-06-2023-0171>

Barnes, M. (2011). *Findings of the inquest into the death of Ryan Charles Saunders* Brisbane: Office of the State Coroner, Queensland Retrieved from <https://www.courts.qld.gov.au/__data/assets/pdf_file/.../cif-saunders-rc-20111007.pdf>

Bennett, J. K., Fuertes, J. N., Keitel, M., & Phillips, R. (2011). The role of patient attachment and working alliance on patient adherence, satisfaction, and health-related quality of life in lupus treatment. *Patient Education and Counseling*, *85*(1), 53–59. <https://doi.org/10.1016/j.pec.2010.08.005>

Berry, J. W. (1997). Immigration, acculturation, and adaptation. *Applied Psychology: An International Journal, 46*, 5–68.

Biquet, J. M., Schopper, D., Sprumont, D., & Michel, P. (2021). A call for the application of patient safety culture in medical humanitarian action: A literature review. *J Patient Saf, 17*(8), e1732–e1737. <https://doi.org/10.1097/PTS.0000000000000638>

Bourhis, R. Y., Roth, S., & MacQueen, G. (1989). Communication in the hospital setting: A survey of medical and everyday language use amongst patients, nurses and doctors. *Social Science and Medicine, 28*, 339–346.

Brann, M., Bute, J., Keeley-Vassberg, M., Petronio, S., Pines, R., & Watson, M. (2021). Interpersonal health communication theories. In Teresa Thompson & P. J. Schulz (Eds.), *Health communication theory* (pp. 68–89). Wiley.

Brattebo, G., & Flaatten, H. K. (2023). Errors in medicine: Punishment versus learning medical adverse events revisited - expanding the frame. *Current Opinion in Anaesthesiology, 36*(2), 240–245. <https://doi.org/10.1097/ACO.0000000000001235>

Brewer, M. B., & Kramer, R. M. (1985). The psychology of intergroup attitudes and behavior. *Annual Review of Psychology, 36*(1), 219–243. <https://doi.org/10.1146/annurev.ps.36.020185.001251>

Burgoon, J. K., Pfau, M., Parrott, R., Birk, T. S., Coker, R., & Burgoon, M. (1987). Relational communicating, satisfaction, compliance-gaining strategies, and compliance in communication between physicians and patients. *Communication Monographs, 54*, 307–324.

Burgoon, M., Parrott, R., Burgoon, J. K., Ciker, R., Pfau, M., & Birk, T. S. (1990). Patients' severity of illness, noncompliance, and locus of control and physicians' compliance-gaining messages. *Health Communication, 1*, 29–46.

Butow, P. N., Sze, M., Eisenbruch, M., Bell, M. L., Aldridge, L. J., Abdo, S., Tanious, M., Dong, S., Iedema, R., Vardy, J., Hui, R., Boyle, F., Liauw, W., & Goldstein, D. (2013). Should culture affect practice? A comparison of prognostic discussions in consultations with immigrant versus native-born cancer patients. *Patient Education and Counseling, 92*(2), 246–252. <https://doi.org/10.1016/j.pec.2013.03.006>

Byrne, D. (1969). Attitudes and attraction. *Advances in Experimental Social Psychology, 4*, 35–89.

Capell, J., Dean, E., & Veenstra, G. (2008). The relationship between cultural competence and ethnocentrism of health care professionals. *Journal of Transcultural Nursing, 19*(2), 121–125. <https://doi.org/10.1177/1043659607312970>

Capella, J. N., & Street, R. L., Jr. (1985). Sequence and pattern in communicative behaviour: A model and commentary. In R. L. Street & J. N. Capella (Eds.), *Sequence and pattern in communicative behaviour.* Edward Arnold.

Cargile, A. C., & Giles, H. (1996). Intercultural communication training: Review, critique, and a new theoretical framework. In B. Burleson (Ed.), *Communication yearbook* (Vol. 19, pp. 385–423).

Cegala, D., McGee, D., & McNeilis, K. (1996). Components of patients' and doctors' perceptions of communication competence during a primary care medical interview. *Health Communication*, *8*(1), 1–27.

Cegala, D. J., & Broz, S. L. (2002). Physician communication skills training: A review of theoretical backgrounds, objectives and skills. *Medical Education*, *36*, 1004–1016.

Cegala, D. J., & Broz, S. L. (2003). Provider and patient communication skills training. In T. L. Thompson, A. Dorsey, R. Parrott, & K. Miller (Eds.), *Handbook of health communication* (pp. 95–119). Routledge. <https://doi.org/10.4324/9781410607683>

Chevalier, B. A., Watson, B. M., Barras, M. A., & Cottrell, W. N. (2016). Hospital pharmacists' perceptions of medication counseling: A focus group study. *Research in Social & Administrative Pharmacy*, *12*(5), 756–771. <https://doi.org/10.1016/j.sapharm.2015.10.007>

Chevalier, B. A. M., Watson, B. M., Barras, M. A., & Cottrell, W. N. (2020). Assessing communication behaviours of hospital pharmacists: How well do the perspectives of pharmacists, patients, and an independent observer align? *Journal of Language and Social Psychology*, *39*(5–6), 626–652. <https://doi.org/10.1177/0261927x20909867>

Chevalier, B. A. M., Watson, B. M., Barras, M. A., Cottrell, W. N., & Angus, D. J. (2018). Using Discursis to enhance the qualitative analysis of hospital pharmacist-patient interactions. *PloS One*, *13*(5). <https://doi.org/10.1371/journal.pone.0197288>

Chevalier, B. A. M., Watson, B. M., Barras, M. l. A., & Cottrell, W. N. (2017). Investigating strategies used by hospital pharmacists to effectively communicate with patients during medication counselling. *Health Expectations*, *20*(5), 1121–1132. <https://doi.org/10.1111/hex.12558>

Chevalier, B. A. M., Watson, B. M., & Cottrell, N. (2020). Pharmacy students' self-reported attitudes, beliefs and behaviors about communicating with patients, measured over time. *Pharmacy Education*, *20*(1), 116–126. <https://doi.org/10.46542/pe>

Clayton, M. F., Parker, P. D., & Ellington, L. (2021). The multiple voices of communication in healthcare. In Teresa L. Thompson & N. G. Harrington (Eds.), *The Routledge handbook of health communication* (Third ed., pp. 229–243). Routledge. <https://doi.org/10.4324/9781003043379>

Convery, S. (2023). *Half of migrant workers in Australia feel unsafe at work, survey finds*. Guardian Media Group. <https://www.theguardian.com/australia-news/2023/mar/20/half-of-migrant-workers-in-australia-feel-unsafe-at-work-survey-finds?CMP=share_btn_url>

Coupland, N., Coupland, J., Giles, H., & Henwood, K. (1988). Accommodating the elderly: Invoking and extending a theory. *Language in Society*, *17*(1), 1–41. <https://doi.org/10.2307/4167896>

Coupland, N., Wiemann, J. M., & Giles, H. (1991). Talk as "problem" and communication as "miscommunication." An integrative analysis. In N. Coupland, H. Giles, & J. M. Wiemann (Eds.), *"Miscommunication" and problematic talk* (pp. 1–17). Sage.

Cronbach, L. R. (1951). Coefficient alpha and the internal structure of tests. *Psychometrika*, *16*, 297–334.

D'Agostino, T. A., & Bylund, C. L. (2011). The nonverbal accommodation analysis system (naas): Initial application and evaluation. *Patient Education and Counseling*, *85*(1), 33–39. <https://doi.org/10.1016/j.pec.2010.07.043>

Dinos, S., Ascoli, M., Owiti, J. A., & Bhui, K. (2017). Assessing explanatory models and health beliefs: An essential but overlooked competency for clinicians. *BJPsych Advances*, *23*(2), 106–114. <https://doi.org/10.1192/apt.bp.114.013680>

Douglas, R. N., Stephens, L. S., Posner, K. L., Davies, J. M., Mincer, S. L., Burden, A. R., & Domino, K. B. (2021). Communication failures contributing to patient injury in anaesthesia malpractice claims. *British Journal of Anaesthesia*, *127*(3), 470–478. <https://doi.org/10.1016/j.bja.2021.05.030>

Du Pre, A., & Cook Overton, B. (2023). *Communicating about health: Current issues and perspectives* (7 ed.) [Health Communication]. Oxford University Press.

Dunbar, J., Reddy, P., & May, S. (2011). *Deadly healthcare*. Australian Academic Press.

Epner, D. E., & Baile, W. F. (2012). Patient-centered care: The key to cultural competence. *Annals of Oncology*, *23*, iii33–iii42. <https://doi.org/10.1093/annonc/mds086>

Ericson, C. A. (2015). *Hazard analysis techniques for system safety*. Wiley. <http://ebookcentral.proquest.com/lib/polyu-ebooks/detail.action?docID=2073475>

Fisher, N. L. (1992). Ethnocultural approaches to genetics. *Pediatric Clinics of North America*, *39*(1), 55–64. <https://doi.org/10.1016/S0031-3955(16)38262-1>

Foronda, C., MacWilliams, B., & McArthur, E. (2016). Interprofessional communication in healthcare: An integrative review. *Nurse Education in Practice*, *19*, 36–40. <https://doi.org/10.1016/j.nepr.2016.04.005>

Freimuth, V. S., Masset, H. A., & Meltzer, W. (2006). A descriptive analysis of 10 years of research published in the journal of health communication. *Journal of Health Communication*, *11*, 11–20.

Frenk, J., Chen, L., Bhutta, Z. A., Cohen, J., Crisp, N., Evans, T., Fineberg, H., Garcia, P., Ke, Y., Kelley, P., Kistnasamy, B., Meleis, A., Naylor, D.,

Pablos-Mendez, A., Reddy, S., Scrimshaw, S., Sepulveda, J., Serwadda, D., & Zurayk, H. (2010). Health professionals for a new century: Transforming education to strengthen health systems in an interdependent world. *The Lancet*, *376*(9756), 1923–1958. <https://doi.org/10.1016/S0140-6736(10)61854-5>

Gallagher, T. H. M. D., Studdert, D. L. L. B. S. M. P. H., & Levinson, W. M. D. (2007). Disclosing harmful medical errors to patients current concepts. *The New England Journal of Medicine*, *356*(26), 2713–2719. <https://doi.org/http://dx.doi.org/10.1056/NEJMra070568>

Gallois, C. (2006). Reconciliation through communication in intercultural encounters: Potential or peril? *Journal of Communication*, *53*(1), 5–15. <https://doi.org/10.1111/j.1460-2466.2003.tb03001.x>

Gallois, C., Giles, H., Jones, E., Cargile, A. C., & Ota, H. (1995). Communication accommodation theory: Elaborations and extensions. In R. Wiseman (Ed.), *Intercultural communication theory* (pp. 115–147). Sage.

Gallois, C., Watson, B. M., & Giles, H. (2018). Intergroup communication: Identities and effective interactions. *Journal of Communication*, *68*(2), 309–317. <https://doi.org/10.1093/joc/jqx016>

Gallois, C., Wilmott, L., White, B., Winch, S., Parker, M., Graves, N., Shepherd, N., & Close, E. (2015). Futile treatment in hospital: Doctors' intergroup language. *Journal of Language and Social Psychology*, *34*(6), 657–671. <https://doi.org/10.1177/0261927x15586430>

Garzon Gonzalez, G., Alonso Safont, T., Zamarron Fraile, E., Canada Dorado, A., Luaces Gayan, A., Conejos Miquel, D., Villanueva Sanz, C., Aguado Arroyo, O., Jurado Balbuena, J. J., Castelo Jurado, M., Magan Tapia, P., Barbera Martin, A., Toribio Vicente, M. J., Drake Canela, M., San Jose Saras, D., & Mediavilla Herrera, I. (2023). Is primary care a patient-safe setting? Prevalence, severity, nature, and causes of adverse events: Numerous and mostly avoidable. *International Journal of Quality of Health Care*, *35*(2). <https://doi.org/10.1093/intqhc/mzad019>

Gasiorek, J., & van de Poel, K. (2012). Divergent perspectives on language-discordant mobile medical professionals' communication with colleagues: An exploratory study. *Journal of Applied Communication Research*, *40*(4), 368–383. <https://doi.org/10.1080/00909882.2012.712708>

Gasiorek, J., Van de Poel, K., & Blockmans, I. (2015). What do you do when you can't accommodate? Managing and evaluating problematic interactions in a multilingual medical environment. *Language & Communication*, *41*, 84–88. <https://doi.org/10.1016/j.langcom.2014.10.005>

Giles, H. (1973). Accent mobility: A model and some data. *Anthropological Linguistics*, *15*(2), 87–105.

Giles, H. (2016). *Communication accommodation theory: Negotiating personal relationships and social identities across contexts* (Vol. null).

Giles, H., Bourhis, R. Y., & Taylor, D. M. (1977). Towards a theory of language in ethnic group relations. In H. Giles (Ed.), *Language, ethnicity and intergroup relations*. Academic Press.

Giles, H., Edwards, A. L., & Walther, J. B. (2023). Communication accommodation theory: Past accomplishments, current trends, and future prospects. *Language Sciences*, *99*, 101571. <https://doi.org/10.1016/j.langsci.2023.101571>

Giles, H., & Jin, D. (2025). Accommodating nursing: A communication perspective. *Nursing and Care Open Access Journal*, *11*(1).

Giles, H., Mulac, A., Bradac, J. J., & Johnson, P. (1987). Speech accommodation theory: The first decade and beyond. In M. McLaughlin (Ed.), *Communication yearbook* (Vol. 10, pp. 13–48). Sage.

Giles, H., & Powesland, P. F. (1975). *Speech style and social evaluation.* Academic Press.

Gudykunst, W. B. (2005). *Theorizing about intercultural communication*. Sage.

Guttman, O. T., Lazzara, E. H., Keebler, J. R., Webster, K. L. W., Gisick, L. M., & Baker, A. L. (2021). Dissecting communication barriers in healthcare: A path to enhancing communication resiliency, reliability, and patient safety. *J Patient Saf*, *17*(8), e1465–e1471. <https://doi.org/10.1097/PTS.0000000000000541>

Haidet, P., O'Malley, K. J., Sharf, B. F., Gladney, A. P., Greisinger, A. J., & Jr, R. L. S. (2008). Characterizing explanatory models of illness in healthcare: Development and validation of the connect instrument. *Patient Education and Counseling*, *73*(2), 232-239. <https://doi.org/http://dx.doi.org/10.1016/j.pec.2008.07.007>

Hall, E. T. (1973). *The silent language*. Anchor Books.

Hanson, J., Walsh, S., Mason, M., Wadsworth, D., Framp, A., & Watson, K. (2020). 'Speaking up for safety': A graded assertiveness intervention for first year nursing students in preparation for clinical placement: Thematic analysis. *Nurse Education Today*, *84*, 104252. <https://doi.org/10.1016/j.nedt.2019.104252>

Harrington, N. G., Francis, D., B., & Occa, A. (2022). Theoretical and methodological matters in health communication. In H. Teresa L. Thompson, Nancy Grant (Ed.), *The Routledge Handbook of Health Communication* (Third edition. ed., pp. 17–32). Routledge.

Heider, F. (1958). *The psychology of interpersonal relations / fritz heider.* Lawrence Erlbaum Associates.

Hewett, D. G., Watson, B. M., & Gallois, C. (2013). Trust, distrust, and communication accommodation among hospital doctors. In C. N. Candlin & J. Crichton (Eds.), *Discourses of trust* (pp. 36–51). Palgrave Macmillan UK. <https://doi.org/10.1007/978-1-137-29556-9_3>

Hewett, D. G., Watson, B. M., Gallois, C., Ward, M., & Leggett, B. A. (2009). Intergroup communication between hospital doctors: Implications for quality of patient care. *Social Science and Medicine*, *69*(12), 1732–1740. <https://doi.org/10.1016/j.socscimed.2009.09.048>

Hogg, M. A. (2015). Constructive leadership across groups: How leaders can combat prejudice and conflict between subgroups. In *Advances in group processes* (Vol. 32, pp. 177–207). Emerald Group Publishing Limited. <https://doi.org/10.1108/S0882-614520150000032007>

Hogg, M. A. (2016). Social identity theory. In S. McKeown, R. Haji, & N. Ferguson (Eds.), *Understanding peace and conflict through social identity theory: Contemporary global perspectives* (pp. 3–17). Springer International Publishing. <https://doi.org/10.1007/978-3-319-29869-6_1>

Hogg, M. A., Van Knippenberg, D., & Rast, I. D. E. (2012). Intergroup leadership in organizations: Leading across group and organizational boundaries [Article]. *Academy of Management Review*, *37*(2), 232–255. <https://doi.org/10.5465/amr.2010.0221>

Homans, G. C. (1961). *Social behavior.* Harcourt, Brace & World.

Horrocks, S., Anderson, E., & Salisbury, C. (2002). Systematic review of whether nurse practitioners working in primary care can provide equivalent care to doctors. *BMJ*, *324*(7341), 819–823. <https://doi.org/10.1136/bmj.324.7341.819>

Hsieh, E. (2006). Understanding medical interpreters: Reconceptualizing bilingual health communication. *Health Communication*, *20*(2), 177–186. <https://doi.org/10.1207/s15327027hc2002_9>

Hsieh, E. (2016). *Bilingual Health Communication: Working with Interpreters in Cross-Cultural Care* (1 ed.). Routledge. https://doi.org/10.4324/97813156 58308

Imran, D., Rog, K., Gallichio, J., & Alston, L. (2021). The challenges of becoming and being a clinician manager: A qualitative exploration of the perception of medical doctors in senior leadership roles at a large Australian health service. *BMC Health Services Research*, *21*(1), 351. <https://doi.org/10.1186/s12913-021-06356-w>

Institute of Medicine Committee on Quality of Health Care in, A. (2000). In L. T. Kohn, J. M. Corrigan, & M. S. Donaldson (Eds.), *To err is human: Building a safer health system*. National Academies Press (US)

Copyright 2000 by the National Academy of Sciences. All rights reserved. <https://doi.org/10.17226/9728>

Isaacs, T., Laurier, M. D., Turner, C. E., & Segalowitz, N. (2011). Identifying second language speech tasks and ability levels for successful nurse oral interaction with patients in a linguistic minority setting: An instrument development project. *Health Communication*, *26*(6), 560–570. <https://doi.org/10.1080/10410236.2011.558336>

Jalal, M., Bardhan, K. D., Sanders, D., & Illing, J. (2019). International: Overseas doctors of the nhs: Migration, transition, challenges and towards resolution. *Future Healthcare Journal*, *6*(1), 76–81. <https://doi.org/10.7861/futurehosp.6-1-76>

The joint commission sentinel events data 2023 annual review. (2024). IL, USA Retrieved from <https://www.jointcommission.org/-/media/tjc/documents/resources/patient-safety-topics/sentinel-event/2024/2024_>

Jones, L., Sheeran, N., Lanyon, H., Evans, K., & Martincovic, T. (2018). Nurses' perceptions of communicating with minority parents in a neonatal nursery: A communication accommodation theory approach. *Journal of Communication in Healthcare*, *11*(3), 175–185. <https://doi.org/10.1080/17538068.2018.1460959>

Jones, L., Sheeran, N., Pines, R., & Saunders, B. (2019). How do health professionals decide whether an interpreter is needed for families in neonatal and pediatric units? *Patient Education and Counseling*, *102*(9), 1629–1635. <https://doi.org/10.1016/j.pec.2019.04.004>

Jones, L., Taylor, T., Watson, B., Fenwick, J., & Dordic, T. (2015). Negotiating care in the special care nursery: Parents' and nurses' perceptions of nurse-parent communication. *Journal of Pediatric Nursing*, *30*(6), e71–80. <https://doi.org/10.1016/j.pedn.2015.03.006>

Jones, L., Watson, B. M., Hobman, E., Bordia, P., Gallois, C., & Callan, V. (2008). Employees' perceptions of organizational change: Impact of hierarchical level,. *Leadership and Organization Development Journal*, *29* (4), 294–316.

Kellogg, K. M., Hettinger, Z., Shah, M., Wears, R. L., Sellers, C. R., Squires, M., & Fairbanks, R. J. (2017). Our current approach to root cause analysis: Is it contributing to our failure to improve patient safety? *BMJ Quality & Safety*, *26*(5), 381. <https://doi.org/10.1136/bmjqs-2016-005991>

Kelly, R. J., & Hearld, L. R. (2020). Burnout and leadership style in behavioral health care: A literature review. *The Journal of Behavioral Health Services & Research*, *47*(4), 581–600. <https://doi.org/10.1007/s11414-019-09679-z>

Kim, Y. Y. (2001). *Becoming intercultural: An integrative theory of communication and cross-cultural adaptation.* Sage.

Kleinman, A. (1978). Concepts and a model for the comparison of medical systems as cultural systems. *Social Science & Medicine. Part B: Medical Anthropology*, *12*, 85–93. <https://doi.org/10.1016/0160-7987(78)90014-5>

Kleinman, A., & Benson, P. (2006). Anthropology in the clinic: The problem of cultural competency and how to fix it. *PLoS Medicine*, *3*(10). <https://doi.org/10.1371/journal.pmed.0030294>

Koch, P. l. E., Simpson, D., Toth, H., Marcdante, K., Densmore, E. D., Young, S., Weisgerber, M., Morzinski, J. A., & Havas, N. (2014). Clinical clerkship students' perceptions of (un)safe transitions for every patient. *Academic Medicine*, *89*(3), 477–481. <https://doi.org/10.1097/ACM.0000000000000153>

Korsch, B. M., Gozzi, E. K., & Francis, V. (1968). Gaps in doctor-patient interaction and patient satisfaction. *Journal of Pediatrics*, *42*, 855–871.

Korsch, B. M., & Negrete, V. F. (1972). Doctor-patient communication. *Scientific American*, *227*, 66–74.

Kwok, Y. T. A., Mah, A. P., & Pang, K. M. (2020). Our first review: An evaluation of effectiveness of root cause analysis recommendations in Hong Kong public hospitals. *BMC Health Services Research*, *20*(1), 507. <https://doi.org/10.1186/s12913-020-05356-6>

Larsen, K. M., & Smith, C. K. (1981). Assessment of nonverbal communication in the patient-physician interview. *The Journal of family practice*, *12*, 481–488.

Leach, L., Hastings, B., Schwarz, G., Watson, B., Bouckenooghe, D., Seoane, L., & Hewett, D. (2021). Distributed leadership in healthcare: Leadership dyads and the promise of improved hospital outcomes. *Leadership in Health Services*, *34*(4), 353–374. <https://doi.org/10.1108/LHS-03-2021-0011>

Leonard, M., Graham, S., & Bonacum, D. (2004). The human factor: The critical importance of effective teamwork and communication in providing safe care. *Quality and Safety in Health Care*, *13*(suppl 1), i85–i90. <https://doi.org/10.1136/qshc.2004.010033>

Ley, P. (1988). *Communicating with patients: Improving communication, satisfaction and compliance.* Croom Helm.

Li, B., Watson, B., & Yung, A. (2025). When medical consultations are not face-to-face: a pilot study of patient-centred care communication during coronavirus disease 2019. *mHealth, 11*, 14. https://doi.org/10.21037/mhealth-24-59.

Lingard, L. (2012). Rethinking competence in the context of teamwork. In B. D. Hodges, L. Lingard, & M. B. Anderson (Eds.), *The question of competence : Reconsidering medical education in the twenty-first century* (pp. 42-69). Cornell University Press.

Lingard, L., Espin, S., Whyte, S., Regehr, G., Baker, G. R., Reznick, R., Bohnen, J., Orser, B., Doran, D., & Grober, E. (2004). Communication failures in the operating room: An observational classification of recurrent types and effects. *Quality and Safety in Health Care*, *13*(5), 330–334.

Lozano, F. (2014). Basic theories of traditional Chinese medicine. In Y.-C. Lin & E. S.-Z. Hsu (Eds.), *Acupuncture for pain management* (pp. 13–43). Springer New York. <https://doi.org/10.1007/978-1-4614-5275-1_2>

Lucian L, L. (2009). Errors in medicine. *Clinica Chimica Acta*, *404*(1), 2–5. <https://doi.org/10.1016/j.cca.2009.03.020>

Maass, A., Salvi, D., Arcuri, L., & Semin, G. (1989). Language use in intergroup contexts: The linguistic intergroup bias. *Journal of Personality and Social Psychology*, *57*, 981–993.

MacIntyre, P., D.,, Clement, R., Dornyei I, Z., & Noels, K., A. (1998). Conceptualizing willingness to communicate in a l2: A situational model of l2 confidence and affiliation. *The Modern Language Journal*, *82*(4), 545-562. <https://doi.org/10.1111/j.1540–4781.1998.tb05543.x>

McCroskey, J. C., & Richmond, V. P. (1987). Willingness to communication. In J. C. McCroskey & J. A. Daly (Eds.), *Personality and interpersonal communication* (pp. 119–131). Sage.

Muñiz-Velázquez, J. A., & Pulido, C. (2018). *The Routledge Handbook of Positive Communication: Contributions of an Emerging Community of Research on Communication for Happiness and Social Change.*

Noble, H., & Heale, R. (2019). Triangulation in research, with examples. *Evidence-Based Nursing, 22*(3), 67–68. <https://doi.org/10.1136/ebnurs-2019-103145>

O'Connor, P., O'Malley, R., Kaud, Y., Pierre, E. S., Dunne, R., Byrne, D., & Lydon, S. (2023). A scoping review of patient safety research carried out in the republic of Ireland. *Irish Journal of Medical Science (1971 -), 192*(1), 1–9. <https://doi.org/10.1007/s11845-022-02930-1>

Olazo, K., Gallagher, T. H., & Sarkar, U. (2023). Experiences and perceptions of healthcare stakeholders in disclosing errors and adverse events to historically marginalized patients. *J Patient Saf, 19*(8), 547–552. <https://doi.org/10.1097/PTS.0000000000001173>

Otten, S. (2016). The minimal group paradigm and its maximal impact in research on social categorization. *Current Opinion in Psychology, 11*, 85–89. <https://doi.org/http://dx.doi.org/10.1016/j.copsyc.2016.06.010>

Panagioti, M., Khan, K., Keers, R., N. , Abuzour, A., Phipps, D., Kontopantelis, E., Bower, P., Campbell, S., Haneef, R., Avery, A., J. , & Ashcroft, D., M. . (2019). Prevalence, severity, and nature of preventable patient harm across medical care settings: Systematic review and meta-analysis. *BMJ, 366*, l4185. <https://doi.org/10.1136/bmj.l4185>

Pandey, M., Maina, R. G., Amoyaw, J., Li, Y., Kamrul, R., Michaels, C. R., & Maroof, R. (2021). Impacts of English language proficiency on healthcare access, use, and outcomes among immigrants: A qualitative study. *BMC Health Services Research, 21*(1), 741. <https://doi.org/10.1186/s12913-021-06750-4>

Pattillo, M., Stieglitz, S., Angoumis, K., & Gottlieb, N. (2023). Racism against racialized migrants in healthcare in Europe: A scoping review. *International Journal for Equity in Health, 22*(1), 201. <https://doi.org/10.1186/s12939-023-02014-1>

Peadon, R., Hurley, J., & Hutchinson, M. (2020). Hierarchy and medical error: Speaking up when witnessing an error. *Safety Science, 125*, 104648. <https://doi.org/10.1016/j.ssci.2020.104648>

Peerally, M. F., Carr, S., Waring, J., & Dixon-Woods, M. (2017). The problem with root cause analysis. *BMJ Qual Saf, 26*(5), 417–422. <https://doi.org/10.1136/bmjqs-2016-005511>

Pendleton, D. (1983). Doctor-patient communication: A review. In D. Pendleton & J. Hasler (Eds.), *Doctor-patient communication* (pp. 5–53). Academic Press, Inc.

Percarpio, K. B., Watts, B. V., & Weeks, W. B. (2008). The effectiveness of root cause analysis: What does the literature tell us? *The Joint Commission Journal on Quality and Patient Safety*, *34*(7), 391–398.

Peterson, M. F., & Castro, S. L. (2006). Measurement metrics at aggregate levels of analysis: Implications for organization culture research and the globe project. *The Leadership Quarterly*, *17*(5), 506–521. <http://www.sciencedirect.com/science/article/B6W5N-4KV3XTY-1/2/e566943e865888de068a51a0969df9ae>

Pines, R., Giles, H., & Watson, B. (2021). Managing patient aggression in healthcare: Initial testing of a communication accommodation theory intervention. *Psychology of Language and Communication*, *25*(1), 62–81. <https://doi.org/doi:10.2478/plc-2021-0004>

Queensland Public Hospitals Commission of Inquiry. (2005). *Queensland public hospitals commission of inquiry* (2). Brisbane: Queensland State Archives.

Rittel, H. W. J., & Webber, M. M. (1973). Dilemmas in a general theory of planning. *Policy Sciences*, *4*(2), 155–169. <https://doi.org/10.1007/BF01405730>

Robertson, E. R., Morgan, L., Bird, S., Catchpole, K., & McCulloch, P. (2014). Interventions employed to improve intrahospital handover: A systematic review. *BMJ Quality & Safety*, *23*(7), 600–607. <https://doi.org/10.1136/bmjqs-2013-002309>

Roter, D., & Larson, S. (2002). The roter interaction analysis system (rias): Utility and flexibility for analysis of medical interactions. *Patient Education and Counseling*, *46*(4), 243–251. <https://doi.org/10.1016/S0738-3991(02)00012-5>

Ruben, B. D. (1990). The health caregiver-patient relationship: Pathology, etiology, treatment. In E. B. Ray & L. Donohew (Eds.), *Communication and health systems and applications.* (pp. 51–68). Lawrence Erlbaum Associates Inc. Publishers.

Ruben, B. D. (1993). What patients remember: A content analysis of critical incidents in health care. *Health Communication*, *5*, 99–112.

Sartini, M., Carbone, A., Demartini, A., Giribone, L., Oliva, M., Spagnolo, A. M., Cremonesi, P., Canale, F., & Cristina, M. L. (2022). Overcrowding in emergency department: Causes, consequences, and solutions—a narrative review. *Healthcare*, *10*(9), 1625. <https://www.mdpi.com/2227-9032/10/9/1625>

Savioli, G., Ceresa, I. F., Gri, N., Bavestrello Piccini, G., Longhitano, Y., Zanza, C., Piccioni, A., Esposito, C., Ricevuti, G., & Bressan, M. A. (2022). Emergency department overcrowding: Understanding the factors to find corresponding solutions. *J Pers Med*, *12*(2). <https://doi.org/10.3390/jpm12020279>

Schinkel, S., Schouten, B. C., Kerpiclik, F., Van Den Putte, B., & Van Weert, J. C. M. (2019). Perceptions of barriers to patient participation: Are they due to language, culture, or discrimination? *Health Communication*, *34*(12), 1469–1481. <https://doi.org/10.1080/10410236.2018.1500431>

Schneider, D. E., & Tucker, R. K. (1992). Measuring communicative satisfaction in doctor-patient relations: The doctor-patient communication inventory. *Health Communication*, *4*, 19–28.

Schouten, B. C., Cox, A., Duran, G., Kerremans, K., Banning, L. K., Lahdidioui, A., van den Muijsenbergh, M., Schinkel, S., Sungur, H., Suurmond, J., Zendedel, R., & Krystallidou, D. (2020). Mitigating language and cultural barriers in healthcare communication: Toward a holistic approach. *Patient Education and Counseling*, *103*(12), 2604–2608. <https://doi.org/10.1016/j.pec.2020.05.001>

Schouten, B. C., Manthey, L., & Scarvaglieri, C. (2023). Teaching intercultural communication skills in healthcare to improve care for culturally and linguistically diverse patients. *Patient Education and Counseling*, *115*, 107890. <https://doi.org/10.1016/j.pec.2023.107890>

Segalowitz, N., & Kehayia, E. (2011). Exploring the determinants of language barriers in health care (lbhc): Toward a research agenda for the language sciences. *The Canadian Modern Language Review / La revue canadienne des langues vivantes*, *67*, 480–507.

Segalowitz, N. S., Doucerain, M. M., Meuter, R. F. I., Zhao, Y., Hocking, J., & Ryder, A. G. (2016). Comprehending adverbs of doubt and certainty in health communication: A multidimensional scaling approach [Methods]. *Frontiers in Psychology*, *7*(558). <https://doi.org/10.3389/fpsyg.2016.00558>

Seligman, M. E. P. (2011). *Flourish: A visionary new understanding of happiness and well-being.* Free Press.

Semin, G. R., & Fiedler, K. (1991). The linguistic category model, its bases, applications, and range. *European Review of Social Psychology*, *2*, 1–30.

Semin, G. R., & Fiedler, K. (1992). Properties of the interpersonal language and attribution. In G. R. Semin & K. Fiedler (Eds.), *Language, interaction and social cognition* (pp. 58–77). Sage.

Sentinel event statistics. <http://www.Jointcommission.Org/sentinel_event.Aspx.>

Setchell, J., Leach, L. E., Watson, B. M., & Hewett, D. G. (2015). Impact of identity on support for new roles in health care: A language inquiry of doctors' commentary. *Journal of Language and Social Psychology*, *34*, 672–686. <https://doi.org/10.1177/0261927x15586793>

Sheeran, N., Jones, L., & Rowe, J. (2013). The relationship between maternal age, communication and supportive relationships in the neonatal nursery for mothers of preterm infants. *Journal of Neonatal Nursing*, *19*(6), 327–336. <https://doi.org/10.1016/j.jnn.2013.01.006>

Specchia, M. L., Cozzolino, M. R., Carini, E., Di Pilla, A., Galletti, C., Ricciardi, W., & Damiani, G. (2021). Leadership styles and nurses' job satisfaction. Results of a systematic review. *International Journal of*

Environmental Research and Public Health, *18*(4), 1552. <https://www.mdpi.com/1660-4601/18/4/1552>

Street Jr, R. L. (1993). Analyzing messages and their outcomes: Questionable assumptions, possible solutions. *Southern Communication Journal*, *58*(2), 85–90. <https://doi.org/10.1080/10417949309372891>

Street, R. L., Jr. (1985). Participant-observer differences in speech evaluation. *Journal of Language and Social Psychology*, *4*, 125–130.

Street, R. L., Jr. (1991). Accommodation in medical consultations. In H. Giles, J. Coupland, & N. Coupland (Eds.), *Contexts of accommodation: Developments in applied sociolinguistics* (pp. 131–156). Cambridge University Press.

Street, R. L., Jr. (1992). Analyzing communication in medical consultations: Do behavioral measures correspond to patients' perceptions? *Medical Care*, *30*(11), 976–988.

Street, R. L., Jr. (1993). Analyzing messages and their outcomes: Questionable assumptions, possible solutions. *Southern Communication Journal*, *48*, 85–90.

Street, R. L., Jr, & Buller, D. B. (1988). Patients' characteristics affecting physician-patient nonverbal communication. *Human Communication Research*, *15*, 60–90.

Street, R. L., Jr, Mulac, A., & Wiemann, J. M. (1988). Speech evaluation differences as a function of perspective (participant and observer) and presentational medium. *Human Communication Research*, *14*, 333–363.

Street, R. L., Jr, & Wiemann, J. M. (1988). Differences in how physicians and patients perceive physicians' relational communication. *The Southern Speech Communication Journal*, *53*, 420–440.

Street, R. L., Jr., & Wiemann, J. M. (1987). Patient satisfaction with physicians' interpersonal involvement, expressiveness, and dominance. *Communication Yearbook*, *10*, 591–612.

Stucky, C. H., Michael Hartmann, J., Yauger, Y. J., Romito, K. J., Bradley, D. F., Baza, G., Lorenz, M. E., House, S. L., Dindinger, R. A., Wymer, J. A., Miller, M. J., & Knight, A. R. (2024). Surgical safety does not happen by accident: Learning from perioperative near miss case studies. *Journal of Perianesthesia Nursing*, *39*(1), 10–15. <https://doi.org/10.1016/j.jopan.2023.06.095>

Sutcliffe, K. M. P., Lewton, E. P. M. P. H., & Rosenthal, M. M. P. (2004). Communication failures: An insidious contributor to medical mishaps. *Academic Medicine Special Theme: Physician - Patient Relationships*, *79*(2), 186–194.

Tajfel, H. (Ed.). (1978). *Interindividual behaviour and intergroup behaviour* (Vol. 14). Academic Press.

Tajfel, H. (1979). Individuals and groups in social psychology. *British Journal of Social Psychology*, *18*, 183–190.

Taylan, C., & Weber, L. T. (2023). "Don't let me be misunderstood": Communication with patients from a different cultural background.

Pediatric Nephrology, *38*(3), 643–649. <https://doi.org/10.1007/s00467-022-05573-7>

Teal, C. R., & Street, R. L. (2009). Critical elements of culturally competent communication in the medical encounter: A review and model. *Social Science and Medicine*, *68*(3), 533–543. <https://doi.org/DOI: 10.1016/j.socscimed.2008.10.015>

Thomas, S. (2007). Nurse-physician collaboration: A comparison of the attitudes of nurses and physicians in the medical-surgical patient care setting. *Medsurg Nursing*, *16*(2), 87–92.

Thompson, T. L., & Harrington, N. G. (2022). *The Routledge Handbook of Health Communication* (Third edition. ed.). Routledge.

Thompson, T. L., & Robinson, J. D. (2021). The basics of health communication theory. In Teresa L. Thompson & P. J. Schulz (Eds.), *Health communication theory* (pp. 3–18). Wiley Blackwell.

Timilsina Bhandari, K. K., Xiao, L. D., & Belan, I. (2015). Job satisfaction of overseas-qualified nurses working in Australian hospitals. *International Nursing Review*, *62*(1), 64–74. <https://doi.org/10.1111/inr.12146>

Torrens, C., Campbell, P., Hoskins, G., Strachan, H., Wells, M., Cunningham, M., Bottone, H., Polson, R., & Maxwell, M. (2020). Barriers and facilitators to the implementation of the advanced nurse practitioner role in primary care settings: A scoping review. *International Journal of Nursing Studies*, *104*, 103443. <https://doi.org/10.1016/j.ijnurstu.2019.103443>

Turnbull, M., & Wu, X. I. (2025). Navigating migration and cancer in Asia: A narrative analysis of stories told by Filipino migrant domestic workers with breast cancer. *Journal of Migration and Health*, *12*, 100337. <https://doi.org/10.1016/j.jmh.2025.100337>

Umberfield, E., Ghaferi, A. A., Krein, S. L., & Manojlovich, M. (2019). Using incident reports to assess communication failures and patient outcomes. *Joint Commission Journal on Quality and Patient Safety*, *45*(6), 406–413. <https://doi.org/10.1016/j.jcjq.2019.02.006>

Vanderford, M. L., Jenks, E. B., & Sharf, B. F. (1997). Exploring patients' experiences as a primary source of meaning. *Health Communication*, *9*, 13–26.

Vogus, T. J., Sutcliffe, K. M., & Weick, K. E. (2010). Doing no harm: Enabling, enacting, and elaborating a culture of safety in health care. *Academy of Management Perspectives*, *24*(4), 60–77. <https://doi.org/10.5465/AMP.2010.55206385>

Vreugdenhil, J., Somra, S., Ket, H., Custers, E. J. F. M., Reinders, M. E., Dobber, J., & Kusurkar, R. A. (2023). Reasoning like a doctor or like a nurse? A systematic integrative review [Review]. *Frontiers in Medicine*, *10*. <https://doi.org/10.3389/fmed.2023.1017783>

Waitzkin, H. (1990). On studying the discourse of medical encounters: A critique of quantitative and qualitative methods and a proposal for reasonable compromise. *Medical Care*, *28*, 473–488.

Wakefield, M. (2000). To err is human: An institute of medicine report. *Professional Psychology: Research and Practice*, *31*(3), 243–244. <https://doi.org/10.1037/h0092814> (Training and Employment of Professional Psychologists)

Wang, X., & Watson, B. M. (2024). Exploring foreign domestic workers' perceived contextual factors that influence their participation in medical consultations: An ecological lens. *Health Communication*, *39*(1), 161–172. <https://doi.org/10.1080/10410236.2022.2162233>

Watson, B. M. (2020). Communication accommodation theory as an intervention tool to improve interprofessional practice in healthcare. In L. Mullany (Ed.), *Professional communication: Consultancy, advocacy, activism* (pp. 169–189). Springer International Publishing. <https://doi.org/10.1007/978-3-030-41668-3_9>

Watson, B. M., & Gallois, C. (1998). Nurturing communication by health professionals toward patients: A communication accommodation theory approach. *Health Communication*, *10*, 343–355. <https://www.tandfonline.com/doi/abs/10.1207/s15327027hc1004_3>

Watson, B. M., & Gallois, C. (1999). Communication accommodation between patients and health professionals: Themes and strategies in satisfying and unsatisfying encounters. *International Journal of Applied Linguistics*, *9*(2), 167–183.

Watson, B. M., & Gallois, C. (2004). Emotional expression as a sociolinguistic strategy: Its importance in medical interactions. In S. H. Ng, C. N. Candlin, & C. Y. Chiu (Eds.), *Language matters: Communication, culture and identity* (pp. 63–84). City University of Hong Kong Press.

Watson, B. M., Heatley, M., Kruske, S. G., & Gallois, C. (2012). An empirical investigation into beliefs about collaborative practice among maternity care providers. *Australian Health Review*, *36*(4), 466–470. <https://doi.org/10.1071/ah11104>

Watson, B. M., Jones, L., & Cretchley, J. (2014). Time as a key topic in health professionals' perceptions of clinical handovers. *Global Qualitative Nursing Research*, *1*, 1–11. <https://doi.org/10.1177/2333393614550162>

Watson, B. M., Jones, L., & Hewett, D. G. (2016). Accommodating health. In H. Giles (Ed.), *Communication accommodation theory : Negotiating personal relationships and social identities across contexts* (pp. 152–168). Cambridge University Press.

Watson, B. M., & Wu, X. I. (2022). Sentinel events and miscommunication what do we know in 2021: A language and social psychology framework. *Health Communication*, 1–10. <https://doi.org/10.1080/10410236.2022.2031451>

White, S. J., Nguyen, A. D., Roger, P., Tse, T., Cartmill, J. A., Hatem, S., & Willcock, S. M. (2024). Tailoring communication practices to support

effective delivery of telehealth in general practice. *BMC Primary Care*, *25*(1), 232. <https://doi.org/10.1186/s12875-024-02441-1>
Whitt, N., Harvey, R., McLeod, G., & Child, S. (2007). How many health professionals does a patient see during an average hospital stay? *New Zealand Medical Journal*, *120*(1253), U2517.
Williams, A., Giles, H., Coupland, N., Dalby, M., & Manasse, H. (1990). The communicative contexts of elderly social support and health: A theoretical approach. *Health Communication*, *2*, 123–143.
Williams, K. N. (2006). Improving outcomes of nursing home interactions. *Research in Nursing and Health*, *29*(2), 121–133. <https://doi.org/10.1002/nur.20117>
Wong, W., Loong, H., Lee, A., Wong, A., Sum, C., Ching, J., Wu, J., & Lin, Z.-x. (2020). Examining patient preferences for integrative Chinese-western colorectal cancer care in Hong Kong. In (pp. 85–105). <https://doi.org/10.1007/978-981-15-4389-0_5>
World Health, O., & Safety, W. H. O. P. (2010). Conceptual framework for the international classification for patient safety version 1.1: final technical report January 2009. In. Geneva: World Health Organization.
World Health Organization. (2010). *Framework for action on interprofessional education and collaborative practice.* <http://www.who.int/hrh/resources/framework_action/en/>
World Health Organization. (2017, 29 March 2017). *Who launches global effort to halve medication-related errors in 5 years.* Retrieved 12 December from <https://www.who.int/news/item/29-03-2017-who-launches-global-effort-to-halve-medication-related-errors-in-5-years>
World Health Organization. (2019a). *Who calls for urgent action to reduce patient harm in healthcare.* Retrieved 10 May from <https://www.who.int/news/item/13-09-2019-who-calls-for-urgent-action-to-reduce-patient-harm-in-healthcare>
World Health Organization. (2019b). *Who global report on traditional and complementary medicine 2019.* World Health Organization. <https://iris.who.int/handle/10665/312342>
World Health Organization. (2023, 11 September 2023). *Fact sheet on patient safety.* Retrieved 03 December from <https://www.who.int/news-room/fact-sheets/detail/patient-safety>
Yurkovich, E., & Smyer, T. (1998). Shift report: A time for learning. *Journal of Nursing Education*, *37*(9), 401–403.
Zhang, M., Moalin, M., & Haenen, G. (2019). Connecting west and east. *International Journal of Molecular Sciences*, *20*(9). <https://doi.org/10.3390/ijms20092333>
Zhao, Y., Segalowitz, N., Voloshyn, A., Chamoux, E., & Ryder, A. G. (2021). Language barriers to healthcare for linguistic minorities: The case of second

language-specific health communication anxiety. *Health Communication*, *36*(3), 334–346. <https://doi.org/10.1080/10410236.2019.1692488>

Ziersch, A., Due, C., & Walsh, M. (2020). Discrimination: A health hazard for people from refugee and asylum-seeking backgrounds resettled in Australia. *BMC Public Health*, *20*(1), 108. <https://doi.org/10.1186/s12889-019-8068-3>

Zimmermann, M., & Jucks, R. (2018). How experts' use of medical technical jargon in different types of online health forums affects perceived information credibility: Randomized experiment with laypersons. *Journal of Medical Internet Research*, *20*(1), e30. <https://doi.org/10.2196/jmir.8346>

Zorn, T. E., Page, D. J., & Cheney, G. (2000). Nuts about change: Multiple perspectives on change-oriented communication in a public sector organization. *Management Communication Quarterly*, *13*, 515–566.

Index

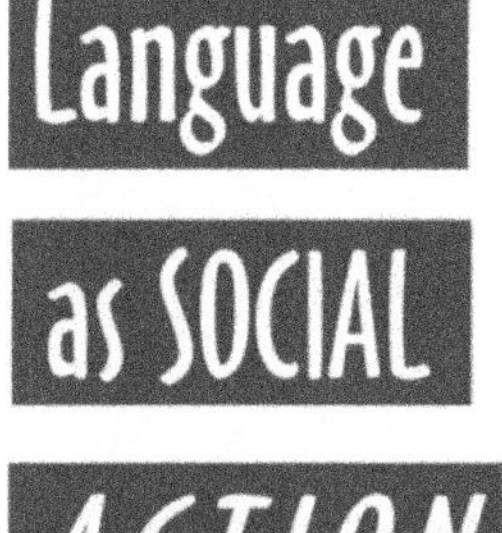
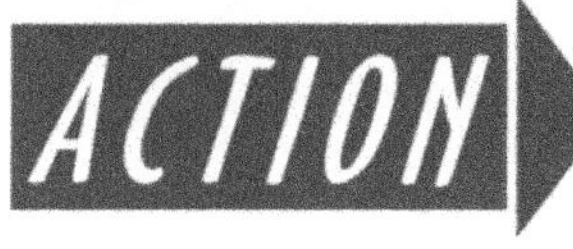

Howard Giles and David M. Markowitz
GENERAL EDITORS

This series explores new and exciting advances in the ways in which language both reflects and fashions social reality—and thereby constitutes critical means of social action. As well as these being central foci in face-to-face interactions across different cultures, they also assume significance in the ways that language functions in the mass media, new technologies, organizations, and social institutions. Language as Social Action does not uphold apartheid against any particular methodological and/or ideological position, but, rather, promotes (wherever possible) cross-fertilization of ideas and empirical data across the many, all-too-contrastive, social scientific approaches to language and communication. Contributors to the series will also accord due attention to the historical, political, and economic forces that contextually bound the ways in which language patterns are analyzed, produced, and received. The series will also provide an important platform for theory-driven works that have profound, and often times provocative, implications for social policy.

For further information about the series and submitting manuscripts, please contact:

Howard Giles
Department of Communication University of California at Santa Barbara Santa Barbara, CA 93106-4020
HowieG iles@cox.net

David M. Markowitz
Department of Communication Michigan State University
East Lansing, MI 48824
dmm@msu.edu

To order other books in this series, please contact our Customer Service Department at:

peterlang@presswarehouse.com (within the U.S.)
orders@peterlang.com (outside the U.S.)

Or browse online by series at:

www.peterlang.com